Outsmarting Mother Nature

Outsmarting Mother Nature

A Woman's Complete Guide to Plastic Surgery

Iliana E. Sweis, MD, FACS

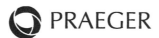 PRAEGER

AN IMPRINT OF ABC-CLIO, LLC
Santa Barbara, California • Denver, Colorado • Oxford, England

Copyright 2010 by IS Devices, LLC

All rights reserved. No part of this publication may be reproduced, stored in a
retrieval system, or transmitted, in any form or by any means, electronic,
mechanical, photocopying, recording, or otherwise, except for the inclusion of
brief quotations in a review, without prior permission in writing from the
publisher.

Library of Congress Cataloging-in-Publication Data

Sweis, Iliana E.
    Outsmarting mother nature : a woman's complete guide to plastic surgery /
Iliana E. Sweis.
        p. cm.
    Includes bibliographical references and index.
    ISBN 978–0–313–38614–5 (hard copy : alk. paper) — ISBN 978–0–313–38615–2
(ebook)
1. Surgery, Plastic—Popular works. I. Title.
RD119.S89   2010
617.9′5—dc22   2009054356

ISBN: 978–0–313–38614–5
EISBN: 978–0–313–38615–2

14 13 12 11 10   1 2 3 4 5

This book is also available on the World Wide Web as an eBook.
Visit www.abc-clio.com for details.

Praeger
An Imprint of ABC-CLIO, LLC

ABC-CLIO, LLC
130 Cremona Drive, P.O. Box 1911
Santa Barbara, California 93116-1911

This book is printed on acid-free paper ∞

Manufactured in the United States of America

My father, Elias Sweis, whose love of art opened my eyes to the beauty that we can create. My mother, Haya Sweis, whose unconditional support gave me the strength and direction to seek my dreams.

My mentors at Northwestern and Case Western Reserve, whose knowledge, guidance and patience allowed me to achieve a most gratifying professional career.

My patients, whose individual experiences and unique perspectives continuously contribute to my understanding of the many dimensions of plastic surgery.

Men fall in love with the women they are attracted to; women become more and more attracted to the men they love.

Anonymous

Contents

Introduction

It is said that beauty is in the eye of the beholder. But does being considered beautiful by others necessarily bring about an inner sense of feeling beautiful? Does how we are perceived by other people control our perception of ourselves? Certainly, there is a significant influence. However, frequently, the opinions that others have about our personal strengths and weaknesses do not reflect what we consider to be our own strengths and weaknesses. If others judge the degree of our personal level of intelligence, thoughtfulness, and etiquette differently than we do, why should we assume that we share their viewpoint regarding our physical appearance? While it is influential, it is not what others believe that sanctions our self-perception, nor is it necessarily what allows us to feel attractive. History is filled with biographies of beautiful women who were devotedly admired because of their external appearance, yet whose personal lives were in shambles. They did not seem prepared for all that society handed to them. Their level of self-confidence and their own sense of beauty never measured up to that which society assumed they deserved, warranted, and possessed. Their stories and our daily observations confirm that being considered beautiful by others is quite different from recognizing one's own physical beauty. These two viewpoints do not always mirror each other. Although we acknowledge that beauty is the eye of the beholder, isn't it just as important (if not more important) for beauty to be in the eye of the beheld?

As women, we are often our own worst critics. We are usually far more judgmental of our physical attributes than men are of theirs, or even of ours. There may or may not be a biological component to this.

However, a significant contributor is the external demands society places on women and their appearance. These are quite different than the types of demands placed on men. Men are assessed by their achievements. The skillful surgeon, the successful stockbroker, the powerful attorney, and the influential businessman are all considered very attractive. Yet, regardless of how successful a woman may be in her career or professional accomplishments, she will also be evaluated by her external appearance. Although this may be perceived as an unfair consequence of society's expectations, to deny it is unrealistic; understandably, it has served to mold women's often overly critical evaluation of their own image.

Women's roles in society and their self-perception have evolved, and continue to evolve, over the course of time. Despite the fact that in the last 50 years, women have become accomplished, successful, influential, and powerful in the workplace, both society and women themselves still demand a great deal of their appearance. When a woman examines a flawlessly airbrushed photograph, either consciously or subconsciously, she compares herself to the image in that photograph. Very few women can view the perfect face in a cosmetic advertisement or the perfectly sculpted and toned body in a fashion magazine and not wish they shared some of the emphasized attributes. A woman will imagine herself with these new and improved features. She will repeatedly ask herself if she would consider making these physical changes. Frequently, she will go back and forth in her decision, changing her mind and dismissing her desire. The progression from wishing she looked a certain way and actually making the decision to undergo changes in her appearance is a huge step, and is the first one that a woman takes before seeking a plastic surgeon.

It is important to understand that when a woman consults with a plastic surgeon to remove the wrinkles from around her eyes, to liposuction her thighs, or to enlarge her breasts, in general she is not being vain. Webster's Dictionary defines vanity as an inflated pride in oneself or one's appearance.[1] In general, when a woman seeks a plastic surgeon, she is not conceited or trying to be better than other women. She simply and truly believes that the smoother eyelids, the slimmer body, or the enhanced breasts will allow her to be like other attractive women, or like she once saw herself. It is very simple. She wants to feel better about herself. If a woman believes that improving one or more of her physical attributes will provide a greater degree of personal comfort, then exploring plastic surgery is a legitimate option. When we truly examine an individual's reasoning for seeking plastic surgery, we begin to realize that plastic surgery has very little to do with vanity. In its purest form, plastic surgery is a means of nourishing an individual's self-esteem. Basically, it allows us to feel more comfortable in our own skin.

Many men seek plastic surgery for the same reasons as women do. They want to remain youthful at many levels. With an average of one pill of Viagra dispensed every 6.3 seconds around the world, men are expecting more out of life, and life is expecting more out of them. They are becoming fathers at later stages of life. They are working professionally well beyond the traditional retirement age of 65. Many men view the physical changes feasible with plastic surgery as not only a means of making them more attractive, but also as a means of making them more competitive in the workforce. Men want to look youthful and fit so that they can compete with the younger men who are strongly permeating the workforce. A man may look older than he feels and want to maintain a strong presence in his field of expertise. He wants to be perceived as more experienced, but he does not want to be perceived as older than his competition. In other words, a man's desire to look better is closely linked to society's perception of a man's attractiveness, a quality significantly impacted by his professional success.

Many more men are beginning to accept and welcome the idea of cosmetic surgery. In the past, many men considered cosmetic surgery, especially facial plastic surgery, to be somewhat effeminate. They had a difficult time dealing with the physical changes after surgery, not just in terms of how they perceived themselves, but also in how others responded to their new image. This is no longer as true. Within the last few years, more men are seeking cosmetic surgery. In fact, according to a review conducted by the American Society for Aesthetic Plastic Surgery (ASAPS), men had 1.1 million cosmetic procedures, accounting for 9 percent of the total cosmetic procedures performed in 2007.[2] The top five most common cosmetic procedures performed on men were liposuction, eyelid surgery, liposuction, breast reduction, and hair transplantation. Although the percentage of cosmetic procedures performed on men dropped from 9 percent in 2007 to 8 percent in 2008,[3] the decrease was unlikely due to a change in how men viewed plastic surgery. The 2008 ASAPS survey indicated that 57 percent of men approved of cosmetic surgery, and 20 percent considered undergoing cosmetic surgery at some point in life.[4] This is not much different from the viewpoint shared by women. The same survey revealed that 56 percent of women approved of cosmetic surgery, and 31 percent considered undergoing a cosmetic surgery procedure. Furthermore, approximately 78 percent of women and 79 percent of men indicated that if they had cosmetic surgery, they would not be embarrassed if people outside of their family and friends knew.[5]

The most likely reason for the slight decrease in the percentage of cosmetic procedures performed on men from 2007 to 2008 was the state of the economy. Although there was an overall 12 percent decrease in the number of cosmetic procedures performed on both men and women, there was a greater impact on the number of procedures performed on men.[6] During that period of time, many men and women were simply unable to allocate funds towards elective procedures. However, in my practice, it was more common for men to postpone undergoing cosmetic procedures since they did not want to take any unnecessary time off work and potentially compromise their jobs.

In general, cosmetic plastic surgery continues to gain a greater acceptance in society as a whole. In 2008, there were nearly 10.3 million cosmetic procedures performed in the United States.[7] Surgical procedures accounted for 17 percent, and non-surgical procedures accounted for the remaining 83 percent of these procedures.[8] Currently, the baby boomers between the ages 35 and 50 account for 46 percent of the total number of cosmetic procedures performed.[9] This segment of the population has contributed greatly to the popularity and wide acceptance of cosmetic surgery. Despite these statistics and greater acceptance of cosmetic surgery as a whole, women continue to far outnumber men in this arena accounting for 91 percent of cosmetic patients in 2007[10] and 92 percent in 2008.[11]

For women, looking better has a tremendous impact on self-esteem because of their own critical evaluation and because of society's expectations. The sense of confidence that allows a woman to emanate grace when she enters a room stems from within her and how she perceives herself. It is not necessarily something that is bestowed upon her by society or by others' admiration. She arrives at this self-actualization by feeling comfortable in her own skin. Many facets of a woman's life contribute to this personal acceptance, including the extent of her accomplishments, the success of her personal and professional relationships, her own recognition of her physical attributes and accolades, and in some cases, the changes achievable with plastic surgery.

The innate desire many women have to improve their physical attributes and the tremendous increase in the acceptance of plastic surgery during the past decade are the two factors that prompted the writing of this book.

Selected Topics for the Plastic Surgery Patient

1

The Thought Process Leading to Cosmetic Surgery

A great deal of soul searching takes place when a woman is willing to undergo surgery in order to change her physical appearance. There are three major reconciliations that she proceeds through at one level or another. The first is to come to terms with the physical aspect of her appearance that concerns her. If she is younger, she will usually present the desire to look similar to others, either her peers or an image created by society. She may think, "I have a terrible profile because of the bump along my nose." "I have always felt inadequate with the size of my breasts." If she is older, she usually presents a longing for something that she has lost. "I always had a flat tummy until I had my third baby." "I used to have nice breasts until I nursed our two children." "I look so tired for my age ... I never had dark circles under my eye before now." "I've been through a very difficult divorce and I've recently noticed the effect it has had on my face." Recognizing the "flaw" or the "change" is the inherent first step that a woman takes towards changing her appearance.

The second step is to overcome the fear of the risks associated with the surgery itself. She begins to think of not only how the improvement would allow her to enhance her features, but also how this may impact other aspects of her life. She contemplates all of the positive aspects of the future surgery, such as making her more attractive to herself and others, boosting her self-esteem, and even giving her the incentive to take better care of herself in terms of diet and exercise. Her desire to change her appearance must be so great that she believes it is worth the risks associated with the surgery itself. In cases in which the patient perceives an actual physical flaw, she often begins to think that any improvement is better than her current physical state. If the physical attribute concerns the patient enough that the fear of an unacceptable cosmetic result does not completely scare her away, she begins making the mental commitment to undergo elective surgery. This is the biggest and most difficult of the three stages in her decision-making process.

The final step in this process occurs when the patient proceeds through several waves of doubt. This occurs after the patient has made the mental commitment to undergo surgery. As she thinks about what she wants to accomplish and actually schedules a consultation with one or several plastic surgeons, she will often say, "What am I doing?" "Do I really want to do this?" There begins to emerge a slight degree or a great degree of doubt. As the consultation day approaches, the doubt becomes greater. This doubt can have many etiologies. It may be due to an underlying guilt she may have about undergoing the procedure. The guilt may stem from the thought that she is doing this without the complete support of her family, or that she is being financially frivolous, or that she is about to change what Mother Nature gave her. A second common cause for doubt stems from the fact that this is elective, yet very real SURGERY, with its many inherent risks. In some cases, the patient begins to question her own sense of what is important. "Am I just being vain?" The underlying reason for this self-doubt is the fact that this surgery is completely elective. There is no medical reason for it. This is not appendicitis, for which not undergoing surgery would lead to severe consequences. In fact, undergoing the cosmetic surgery has the potential to result in severe consequences. But because it is elective, we feel that we have to justify it. Women go through this justification process multiple times before they are ready to discuss the procedure with a plastic surgeon.

When she meets with a plastic surgeon for the first time, the woman can be very vulnerable. She is presenting to a complete stranger that particular part of her face or body that she finds most concerning or unattractive. She is asking for that surgeon's undivided attention, criticism, support, and, subconsciously, compassion. She may reveal her vulnerability by saying, "Do you see many other women who are like this?" This tends to be more true of areas such as breast surgery or liposuction than it is with facial rejuvenation procedures. After all, everyone ages, but not all women have disproportionately small breasts or large thighs. It is this feeling of inadequacy that must be understood and gently treated by the surgeon. Failing to support a woman while in this state or making her feel less attractive is an unfortunate ability of some physicians who find an all-too-receptive audience in a vulnerable patient. If a plastic surgeon offers a procedure that the patient did not solicit or was not considering prior to her consultation, the patient owes it to herself to seek a second or even third opinion.

If the woman feels that she has established a good rapport with the surgeon, she may be more encouraged to undergo surgery. Once she has left the plastic surgeon's office, she may discuss what she has learned with her family or close friends. If she receives positive feedback, she will most likely return to the plastic surgeon's office for additional information or see another plastic surgeon for further input. If she does not receive this positive feedback, she will begin to question her decision all over again. Most patients have decided whether or not to undergo surgery by the time they have left the plastic surgeon's office after their first consultation. In these cases, future hesitations usually diminish with time.

Once a woman has decided to have cosmetic surgery, she will once again begin to question her decision as the surgery date approaches. She will once again proceed through the justification process. This is normal. After all, she is about to undergo elective surgery with all its inherent risks. There are risks to surgery, risks to anesthesia, and risks that the final outcome may not measure up to her expected goals.

By the time a woman actually enters the operating room, she has played that scene numerous times in her mind. She may have thought of how she will be dressed, what the surgeon will say to her, how she will appear when she emerges from the operating room, and finally, how she will appear after the bandages are removed. The last of these is the most critical, and the one over which the surgeon has the least control. As surgeons, we have a certain degree of control over what is surgically accomplished with every procedure, but we have very little control over what the patient thinks we can accomplish with every procedure. The plastic surgeon's discussion prior to surgery is extremely crucial to influencing the expectations the patient will have after surgery.

It is very common for patients to go through a slight depression after elective surgery. It is easy to understand this depression. Imagine having a face lift. For the first few days, the medications have kept you sleepy. After the initial days, you look in the mirror. What is staring at you is not your old face. It isn't even a nice face. It is bruised, swollen, and maybe even asymmetrical. You suddenly think, "My old face wasn't so bad. What possessed me to do this?" "I'll never look normal again." The worst part is that you chose to do this. There wasn't a disease that required treatment. This was completely elective. You chose the procedure, and you chose the surgeon. You feel that you are responsible for all of it. Because of this, most women feel that they cannot voice their concern to their family members.

Frequently, the source of this depression is the patient's lack of awareness of the changes to expect immediately after surgery. Even though they may have been adequately informed of these changes, they may not recall all of them. It is very easy to have selective memory, since patients have a great deal of information to learn prior to the surgery; and frequently, this is overshadowed by a sense of excitement and some anxiety. Generally, if patients truly understand prior to surgery that their appearance will get worse (sometimes much worse) before it gets better, they can tolerate the recovery with a bit more grace. But even with the most well-informed, prepared, and knowledgeable patient, depression during this stage is not totally unexpected.

The depression after surgery may also be due to losing a sense of control. This is seen in both the female and the male patient, but it is especially true in the male patient. Usually a man has control in his daily routine, whether in the workplace or at home. The recovery phase is not under his control. Although women are generally some-what more tolerant of their convalescence, they also feel a lack of con-trol. Both the patient and the surgeon have limited influence over the usual developments and time course of the healing phase. Patients will often ask what to do in order to allow an improved healing phase. Although plastic surgeons prescribe a full postoperative regimen for their patients, the greatest requirement during the healing phase is patience. This applies to the patient as well as to the surgeon. At the early postoperative stage, reassurance is usually the best treatment. If it were possible, I would have my patients avoid looking in the mirror during the entire healing phase. Realistically, patients will scruti-nize every inch of the area that underwent surgery to an exponentially greater extent than prior to surgery. It is important to remember that this is a very normal part of the healing process and is experienced by most patients.

Another source of the depression may also be due to all of the reasons why the patient had doubts prior to surgery. During this convalescent period, she is unable to do much more than rest. Conse-quently, she has a lot of time to think, and all those old thoughts of doubt and guilt resurface. Over the next several days to weeks, as the swelling and bruising subside, she begins to feel somewhat better. As the swelling subsides, she begins looking in the mirror, and she actually begins to recognize and even may like what she sees. But the recovery phase is a process, just like the preparation for surgery. If a patient understands this prior to surgery, the recovery is much easier. It is usually when the patient returns to her daily routine and puts on her makeup or dresses up that she appreciates the transformation that has taken place.

The most serious source of depression may be due to the patient having unrealistic expectations prior to surgery. It is the responsibility of the surgeon to discover this type of patient and to try to explain the realistic and achievable goals of surgery. The surgeon should try to do this, but only once or twice. If the patient continues to have unrealistic expectations or repeatedly asks the same questions, she is not a candidate for an elective procedure. The patient who continues to ask the same question without listening to the answer is, in essence, seeking a different answer from the one provided. She does not like the answer that she is hearing. She wants the plastic surgeon to give a different response. In other words, she wants a different result from what the surgeon is predicting for her, and may be asking for something that is not achievable. This is a dangerous scenario. She needs to step back and reconsider her goals with surgery. If she proceeds with surgery without coming to terms with the realistic potential, it will most certainly be a source of great depression after surgery, and she will not be happy with the eventual outcome.

It is far better not to undergo an elective procedure with its inherent risks, costs, and recovery than to find yourself unhappy with the eventual outcome. It may be said that in life, happiness is an equation of reality divided by expectations; the higher the ratio, the greater the happiness.

$$\text{HAPPINESS} = \frac{\text{REALITY}}{\text{EXPECTATIONS}}$$

If the expectations are much greater than reality, there will be very little happiness. This is just as true of plastic surgery as it is of everything else in life. It is intended as advice and caution to the future patient.

Finally, any woman who undergoes elective surgery with the goal of pleasing someone else will meet with an unhappiness that few can imagine. In my first year of practice, I had the opportunity to meet a very bright and attractive woman who wanted a breast augmentation. She was a successful physician in her 40s who exercised regularly and was in excellent physical shape. Upon examination, it appeared that she would benefit from breast implants. She wore a small B-cup brassiere and elected to become a healthy C cup. We discussed the size and her options on two occasions before making the final decision to create a C cup.

On the day of surgery, she arrived and was very excited about her procedure. She informed me that I would meet her husband when he arrived to pick her up. She tolerated her procedure very well. After surgery, her husband arrived to take her home. Upon his first glance at his wife in the recovery room, he turned to me and said, "What did you do to my wife?" I was stunned. I honestly did not know what he meant. Being very confused at that moment, I explained that I had just performed a breast augmentation on his wife. He looked at me and said "She is too big and for the record, I am very angry." The patient's chest was wrapped with extensive dressings and bandages, and nothing was adequately visible. Obviously, it was impossible to see the actual size or results of the surgery immediately in the recovery room.

During the visits after surgery, the patient came without her husband. Eventually, and reluctantly, I asked her about her husband's reaction in the recovery room. She explained that her husband had been having an affair with a woman who worked for him. His mistress was younger and had breast implants. My patient underwent the surgery hoping the results would impact her husband's behavior. Furthermore, she described her husband as a domineering man who made most of the decisions in their marriage. She was obviously very influenced by his behavior and opinion. Although any objective observer would have seen the significant improvement following her surgery, she could not see it since the one person she wanted to please most did not like the change.

Several months later, my patient confided that she did not discuss her decision to undergo a breast augmentation with her husband until the day of surgery and chose me as her surgeon without his knowledge. Her reaction to his love affair was to exert control in the marriage by making these two major decisions without her husband's input. The final outcome of the surgery was going to be seen as it relates to all of the other issues in their marriage. The result was not going to be perceived in the same fashion as if she had undergone the procedure simply to enlarge her breasts.

Regardless of the result, her husband was not going to be pleased because he did not make the decisions. With such an intimate part of a woman's body as her breasts, his input was very crucial to how she would perceive herself. The underlying marital issues compromised the patient's perception of her surgical results.

No woman should repeat that scenario. Before surgery, a woman needs to think long and hard to discover the underlying reason why she is having the procedure. She must believe that if the final outcome does not please anyone but herself, she will still be happy.

Only at that point can she be certain she is undergoing the surgery for the right reasons. If a woman proceeds with surgery for the right reasons and has realistic expectations, and the surgery meets with her expectations, she will see a magnificent transformation. She will emerge from this metamorphosis into a more beautiful self and experience a pleasure that many others can only imagine. It is my sincerest wish that plastic surgery patients understand all of the possible ramifications of their decisions so that they may experience this fulfillment.

2

Beauty in History and Its Social Impact

The importance of physical beauty has been recognized throughout time. Aristotle (384–322 BC) stated, "Personal beauty is a greater recommendation than any letter of reference." When Aristotle was asked why people desire physical beauty, he responded: "No one who is not blind could ask that question."[1]

From a young age, we are taught to appreciate beauty. Children's fairy tales depict the "beautiful princess" and the "ugly witch." Cinderella was beautiful and kind, but her ugly stepsisters were cruel and malicious. Over time, these childhood fairy tales are replaced with the social icons recognized for their beauty. An icon is defined as anything devotedly admired.[2] These are the faces and individuals whose images are constantly captured by the media for our appreciation and admiration. When we examine these social icons, we learn a great deal about what our society considers attractive.

Many psychological studies have attempted to understand the role that physical appearances play in how people are perceived. In repeated psychological analyses, men and women were shown photographs of attractive and unattractive individuals and asked to evaluate these individuals with respect to their possible personality and professional traits. None of the evaluators received any personal information about the individuals in the photographs. Their assessments were based on each individual's external appearance alone. Unanimously, those who were attractive were judged to be nicer, more successful, and thought to have more friends than the less attractive individuals.[3]

In her book, *Survival of the Prettiest: The Science of Beauty*,[4] Nancy Etcoff notes that attractive people are treated better by society as a whole. This begins early in life. In hospital nurseries, attractive babies are given more attention than their more plain counterparts. In the playground setting, attractive children have more friends than those considered unattractive. Later on, attractive adults are often pampered, forgiven for wrongdoings, and more likely to be favored in daily situations. They are far more likely to get away with things like cheating on exams, traffic tickets, or shoplifting. We like to treat them well with no expectation of a reciprocal gesture. Why do we respond to beautiful people in this fashion?

Etcoff believes that these are intrinsic hard-wired biological responses to good looks that drive many important interpersonal relationships.[5] At a more basic level, there may be a subconscious and primitive reason as to why we seek attractive people. Are we subconsciously thinking of a healthy and beautiful gene pool? The symmetrical bone structure, the strong male physique, and the smooth feminine curves all represent healthy internal structures in a potential mate. The external attractiveness, therefore, implies that the individual will be a suitable mate for propagating our genes. Is it really so basic? Is it simply innate in our genetic makeup? Are we always subconsciously evaluating and selecting the fittest in our culture to produce better offspring? That may be the case in being attracted to the opposite sex, but it does not explain appreciating attractiveness in individuals of the same gender. Is it possible that we learn to appreciate beauty in people just as we learn to appreciate other finer things in life?

Whatever the reason, we are drawn to attractive people. Their physical qualities represent an ideal to which we gravitate. Whether it is because the human eye appreciates beauty, or whether it is a primitive tendency, or because we, like the described study subjects, read more into beauty than meets the eye, the fact remains that beautiful people are more likely to capture our attention than the average person. They may not necessarily keep our attention, but they certainly capture it.

The perception of beauty has changed tremendously throughout history. In the seventeenth century, Sir Peter Paul Rubens painted the beautiful female form as a voluptuous and rather obese character. At that time, beauty was associated with wealth. The upper class could afford to eat well and to excess, while the lower class had limited means for food. Consequently, the full figure was associated with the desirable and wealthy upper class, and as such became the attractive shape.

Today, when a woman describes herself as "Rubenesque," she is not usually being complimentary. The perception of beauty has changed not simply over the course of lengthy centuries, but over the course of decades. Our society has come to admire the svelte shape far more often than in the past. In the 1940s and 1950s, the hourglass shape of Marilyn Monroe was the envy of most women. Over the subsequent five decades, a thinner physique became appreciated.

By the latter end of the twentieth century, not only did women aim to be thin, but also they had to manifest a more sculpted athletic shape. This trend was inevitable as women developed a healthier attitude toward their diet and exercise. Additionally, as they secured more successful roles in professional fields, they were financially able to allocate income towards their bodies. They joined health clubs, hired personal trainers, and adopted specialized diets. This trend also paralleled the role women play in society. As women who traditionally played the role of "housewives" and "mothers" and became more of men's "companions" or "partners," they began to participate more in traditionally male activities. Women became more involved in athletics and consequently, the desired physical appearance became less voluptuous and more toned or even muscular.

Interestingly, unlike the desirable shape for women, the desirable shape for men has not changed over time. One only has to view depictions of the early Greek Olympiads and Michelangelo's David to recognize that the features we admire today in an attractive male physique are the same features admired centuries ago. We admire a youthful and muscular build. A man's other physical features may be important, but they pale by comparison.

The desire for a more athletic shape has influenced the type of plastic surgery procedures that women are seeking in the twenty-first century. With some exceptions, when a woman presents for a breast augmentation, she usually requests a size that is compatible with the rest of her shape. She does not want to be too obvious. She wants something that will complement her figure, not overcome it. Most professional women today want to be able to wear business attire and not have their breasts be the entire focus of attention. They want to be taken seriously and view excessively large breasts as potentially distracting or taking away from their credibility. In addition, very large breasts may have a tendency to make a woman look top-heavy or matronly. Consequently, when a woman wants to maintain a more athletic and slim physique, she will choose an implant that complements and is in proportion with the rest of her figure. This attitude has influenced the opinions of a significant number of women who now desire to replace their current large breast implants with smaller ones.

Breasts are not only part of a woman's body, but they help define her sexuality. Consequently, more than any other body procedure in plastic surgery, breast enhancement needs to be treated with delicateness. If a woman is not involved in a relationship, she will be the only one initially evaluating the results of her surgery. If she is in a long-term relationship, she will perceive the results of surgery through not only her eyes, but also the eyes of her significant other. As such, it is important that the spouse or partner be involved in the discussions before surgery. Although the final decision must be made by the patient, the final outcome will affect both people, and consequently, both need to participate in the dialogue and decision. However, it is crucial for both individuals in the relationship to recognize that the woman's decision is ultimately the right one.

The other procedure that has been also affected by society's trend to appreciate the athletic shape is liposuction. At an obvious level, women want to be thinner. However, it isn't simply a desire to be thinner as much as it is a desire to change their shape. Many women now seek very gradual and straighter hips. As stated previously, the hourglass shape, consisting of the small waist and voluptuous breasts and hips, is not considered as much of an ideal for many women as it may have been in the past. That is not to say that women want masculine bodies, but they do not want extremes. The streamlined body with very smooth, subtle, and gradual curves is the desired feminine body of the twenty-first century. One only has to look at the fashion world to confirm this. Diet and exercise will change one's size, but not one's shape. Liposuction will allow a change in both one's size and one's shape.

The change in the definition of beauty is not just limited to the body. Our perception of the attractive face has also changed. Once again, the trend has been to replace extremes with more natural and more youthful expressions. The three areas that have undergone the most change in this respect are the brow, the nose, and the lips.

The ideal female brow is one that is slightly arched laterally. The exotic and high-arched eyebrows sported by twentieth-century beauties like Joan Collins are still considered beautiful, but have been somewhat replaced with more subtle features. In general, women have become more specific in their demand for a youthful brow and forehead. They want smooth foreheads and slightly arched brows, but they are uncomfortable with extremes. The fear of looking startled or constantly surprised has led many women to be cautious with brow surgery. This has contributed tremendously to the popularity of less aggressive procedures, such as Botox Cosmetic to treat forehead wrinkles, and temporal lifts to treat the lateral brow.

As surgeons became more sophisticated with the techniques available for nasal surgery, patients became more sophisticated in their desire for nasal enhancement. Patients do not want to look like they have had a "nose job." The small and pinched nose popular in the 1970s has been replaced with a more natural nose that suits the other facial features. Frequently, patients will seek a nose that is only slightly different than their existing one. They do not want to look different. They simply want to look better and have a more harmonious nose. The extremes of nasal surgery that have been seen on the faces of our culture's celebrities are viewed by most as being harsh and freakish. Today, ideal nasal surgery creates subtle yet definite refinements that do not always produce such drastic changes.

The lips have also become a focus of attention. Although it has been taken to an extreme by some, fuller lips are now considered very desirable. It is easy to understand this trend. As the face ages, the lips usually become thinner, eventually leading to wrinkles around the lips. When we look at a child's face, we see the smooth skin and the full pouting lips. Full lips are a subconscious image of youth. If a woman does nothing to her face but simply enhances her lips, suddenly she looks younger and more attractive due to the softer, more approachable features. This concept was recognized in ancient times. One only needs to look at the drawings of Cleopatra to appreciate the importance given to full lips as far back as 30 BC. Over 2,000 years later, the trend for many cultures is still to emphasize the lips.

As our criteria for beauty change, and as our roles in society change, so do our personal goals for our appearance. Men and women of the twenty-first century place great demands on themselves professionally and physically. Often, women are overly critical of their flaws because despite the many hurdles they have overcome, they are frequently judged by their external appearance. If a woman has many accomplishments, she will be perceived as yet more successful if she is also attractive. If very successful, a man will be perceived as attractive regardless of his appearance. In today's atmosphere of political correctness, it is difficult to admit this bias, but to deny it is to ignore reality.

3

Changes Occurring within the Face and Body over Time

The human eye appreciates symmetry and harmony. Although no one has a perfectly symmetrical face or body, we usually do not perceive the subtle inherent asymmetry in the human form. However, we quickly recognize more obvious asymmetry. It becomes distracting. It also upsets our sense of beauty when there is incongruity to the face. A disproportionately large nose or small jaw can subconsciously distract our attention from the remaining attractive features within the face.

An attractive face may be likened to a fine architectural design. There needs to be adequate symmetry, projection, and a sense of balance. There are certain relationships and measurements within the face that are thought to portray a more attractive appearance.

In women, a beautiful face starts with a large, smooth forehead, a slightly arched brow, wide-set, large eyes, smooth upper eyelid and distinct lid crease, full eyelashes, prominent cheekbones, a slender sculpted nose, well-defined full lips, and a heart-shaped taper to the jawline. Conversely, the ideal male face has a horizontal brow with very little or no arch, deep-set eyes, a wider nose and mouth, and a squared jawline with prominent muscular definition. Interestingly, the facial aging process leads to a more masculine appearance in both men and women.

Over time, there are many changes in the tissues of the face that lead to the visible signs of aging. These changes affect not only each facial structure, but the proportions of these structures to one another. In addition to the wrinkles and folds that develop over time, as we age, we can expect the following changes to our face:

Loss of fat throughout the face

Subtle receding of the facial bones

Thinning of the lips

Thinning of the skin due to loss of collagen

Drooping of the nasal tip

Enlargement of the earlobes

The loss of fat and receding facial bones result in a loss of adequate support to the skin. This, in combination with the effects of gravity, leads to drooping of the facial tissues. These changes commonly present as jowls and redundancy along the neck. They may also manifest as deep folds that emanate from the side of the nose down toward the lateral side of the mouth (nasolabial folds). The cheek fullness drops slightly below the cheekbone. As the cheek begins to drop, the corners of the mouth turn downward.

The thinning of the skin leads to the very fine wrinkles that develop at the superficial surface of the skin. These are initially most notable along the eyelids. When the thinning of the skin is combined with loss of fat within the soft tissues and thinning of the lips, fine wrinkles develop around the mouth. If an individual has thin skin to begin with, a generalized pattern of superficial wrinkles develops along the entire face, not just the areas around the eyes and mouth.

Over time, most women will see undesirable changes within their bodies. We have to remember that the aging process that occurs within the face is also occurring within the rest of the body. Even the most physically fit women will begin to experience laxity of the skin as the levels of elastin and collagen decrease. With the decreasing estrogen levels, the skin loses some of its elasticity and becomes relaxed. This redundancy leads to folds and wrinkles throughout the body. Early on, the laxity is most visible in the areas where the skin is relatively thin. These are the neck, inner thighs, and upper inner arms. This leads to redundant skin along the neck, rippling along the inner thighs, and flabbiness along the upper inner arms. These three changes occur at relatively the same time. They may be preceded or accompanied by loss of some of the breast tissue, leading to sagging of the breasts. Eventually, the same changes occur within the remaining skin of the abdomen and back. Even thin women will notice that the tight skin above the level of the navel has become lax and redundant. The lax skin and soft tissues along the back become noticeable as a roll over the bra straps. There tends to be an increase in the abdominal girth, leading to a fuller appearance. All of these changes are a natural result of time and the shifting hormone levels women endure.

If Mother Nature adds the effects of childbearing, there are additional expectations. Under most circumstances, childbearing has a tremendous impact on a woman's body. The changes that take place can be unforgiving, from the loss of breast tissue and laxity of the abdomen with stretch marks throughout the body. The stretch marks are usually concentrated over the abdomen, hips, and thighs but may also appear along the breasts. Some women are very fortunate with minimal changes in their bodies following even multiple births. However, for most women, having more than one child is associated with some degree of these compromising changes.

FACIAL REJUVENATION SURGERY: MAINTENANCE VERSUS REVISION

These changes in our faces and bodies are due to many etiologies. There are unavoidable factors, such as aging, gravity, ethnicity, expressiveness, and genetic makeup. There are avoidable factors, such as sun exposure, nicotine exposure, and weight fluctuations. Often, we do not recognize the changes occurring in our face or body until the point at which they are ready for surgical intervention. Usually, a woman will say, "I did not realize that I looked like this until I saw a recent photograph." "When did this happen?" Well, it did not occur overnight, although that is certainly how it may be perceived. The changes have been occurring second by second, minute by minute, day by day. The accumulation of these subtle yet constant changes results in the visible signs of aging.

Women will often ask at what age or time in life should they consider undergoing a face lift or eyelid rejuvenation. There is no single answer to this question. There are two schools of thought regarding facial rejuvenation surgery. One opinion, an older concept, is that a woman should wait until she wants to rejuvenate her eyes, neck, and jowls prior to considering any type of rejuvenation surgery. In other words, she should wait until everything needs to be addressed prior to considering surgery. The other and more accepted school of thought is more of a maintenance regimen. Most plastic surgeons and patients favor this later approach.

More and more women are presenting for surgery at a younger age so that they maintain their youthful appearance and always look rejuvenated. They do not want to appear older and then younger. They want to always look their best and always look natural. In addition, they do not want to undergo a dramatic procedure, experience a dramatic recovery, and have a dramatic change. The maintenance approach has been embraced by patients as they have become more sophisticated in their desires, and it is based on the premise that the less we do surgically, the fewer the facial changes and the more natural the final result.

Most patients seeking facial plastic surgery do not want to look different; they simply want to look more rejuvenated and refreshed. They usually do not want anyone outside of their closest family members or friends to know that they have had anything done. If we take this gradual maintenance approach, there is a certain sequence that most women proceed through for facial rejuvenation.

Usually, the first signs of aging in the face involve the tissues around the eyes, more specifically the drooping of the upper eyelids, the puffiness of the lower eyelids, and the wrinkles around the eyes. Patients will often complain of looking tired all the time. Friends may comment that they look sad, or that they look like they have not had enough rest. Usually, this is due to drooping of the skin in the upper eyelid and wrinkling of the skin of the lower eyelids. In addition, there are normal pockets of fat in both the upper and lower lids that normally help support our eye. With age, or due to heredity and some thyroid disorders, these fat pockets fall forward, giving the appearance of puffiness around the eyes. There is often excess skin along the upper eyelids. The smiles generated through the first three to four decades of life lead to crow's feet along the corners of the eyes. In some circumstances, these changes are accompanied by drooping of the lateral brow. Surgical correction may be performed for either the upper eyelids or the lower eyelids alone, or more commonly for the upper and lower eyelids together. The changes in the brow may be addressed with a brow lift, and the wrinkles around the eyes may be addressed with Botox Cosmetic or laser resurfacing.

The changes continue along the rest of the face, especially notable along the nasolabial folds, the jawline (jowls), and the neck. The relaxation of the skin and soft tissues leads to contour changes most obvious along the lower two-thirds of the face. They manifest as loss of definition along the jawline and less fullness at the level of the cheekbones. It appears as if the cheek soft tissues have dropped from the cheekbone and jawbone. These changes alter the overall shape of the face, replacing the youthful triangular or oval contour with more of a rectangular outline.

Although the age-related changes that take place in the body are more varied than those that occur in the face, there are certain predictable patterns. The greater weight fluctuations one endures, the greater the relaxation of the tissues. The more sun exposure one experiences, the greater the wrinkles along the superficial aspect of the skin. The less the muscle tone and definition one has within the body, the less supporting structures for the overlying skin.

As one would expect, if a woman maintained a very stable weight, exercised regularly to develop a good muscle tone throughout her life, and protected her skin from the sun, she can expect her body to age better. However, even with the most fit and sun-deprived individuals, there are expected changes within the skin. In general, thinner skin ages first. Thin skin is present along the inner thighs and inner upper arms. These areas seem to develop laxity first. Ideally, women would take a proactive approach during their exercise routine very early in life *prior to the development of this laxity* in order to increase muscle tone and provide better support for these areas of thin skin over time.

4

Body Dysmorphic Disorder

It can be said that embarking on plastic surgery is very much like embarking on a love affair. Although it is a little scary at first, it is very exciting. There are emotional roller coasters, there is uncertainty, and there is the hope of possessing the object of one's desires and experiencing happiness only imagined previously. It can also be said that any fool can start a love affair, but it takes a genius to know when it is time to end one. The same may be said of plastic surgery.

When a patient undergoes a long-awaited procedure and has a positive result, she begins to realize that corrective measures may be applied to other parts of her face or body. It is only natural to do so. If plastic surgery can take 10 years away from her face, maybe it can do the same for her thighs or breasts. She is bound to find another part of her face or body that does not suit her more rejuvenated self. Certainly, at times, it is appropriate to enhance other parts of the face or body to complement the overall picture. If the eyes have been lifted, perhaps her neckline now seems relatively older. If the abdomen has undergone liposuction, perhaps her thighs now seem out of proportion with the rest of her shape. But when does seeking additional plastic surgery shift from the normal desire to look better to the compulsive need to achieve perfection?

This is not a question permitting a single answer. In an era when we are encouraged to pursue perfection in every realm of our life, it is very difficult to stop seeking what we perceive to be better. This drive is a natural human tendency, since the human mind is programmed to desire. Once one desire is fulfilled, a new desire is launched. It is only human. It is impossible to satisfy all of our desires because, theoretically, there are an infinite number of these. As long as the desire to achieve a certain goal in plastic surgery is realistic and does not become disruptive or destructive in the individual's life, then it is acceptable.

With that in mind, there is a condition known as Body Dysmorphic Disorder (BDD). It is a condition in which an individual becomes preoccupied with a slight or imagined defect in their appearance. It usually begins during adolescence. Those with BDD focus on a physical flaw to the point that it consumes their daily life. If a slight abnormality is present, the individual magnifies it. The concern is out of proportion to the abnormality. The preoccupation causes a clinically significant negative impact on multiple aspects of the individual's life. It affects their personal, social, and occupational functioning. It can be crippling. In order for the symptoms to be diagnosed as BDD, the individual's preoccupation with the defect must not be accounted for by another mental disorder.

In her book, *The Broken Mirror: Understanding and Treating Body Dysmorphic Disorder*, Katherine Phillips, MD, has identified three patterns of BDD.[1] The first pattern is the most common (40%) and is characterized by preoccupation with one body part over the course of the disorder. In the second pattern (37%), individuals are preoccupied with one body part and add new parts over time, with continuation of their previous concerns. In the third and least common pattern (21%), the preoccupation with one or more body parts disappears and is replaced with new concerns.[2]

Often, patients with BDD will attempt to correct each of the perceived slight or imagined flaws. These flaws become the center of their lives, and all of their energy is spent on finding the surgery that will correct the flaw. Many will stop at no end to achieve their goal. They will travel all over the world to find "the" plastic surgeon who specializes in the procedure that they are seeking. They will undergo six, seven, or maybe more of the same procedure to obtain the "perfect" correction. They will see flaws that no one else would ever notice. More importantly, they will not see the correction achieved with the surgery. They will focus only on the way the surgery fell short of achieving their desired outcome, however slight that may be.

Fortunately, the incidence of BDD is very low in patients seeking elective plastic surgery. David B. Sarwer, PhD, assistant professor of psychology in psychiatry and surgery at the University of Pennsylvania Medical Center, developed a survey to determine the level of experience ASAPS (the American Society of Aesthetic Plastic Surgery) members have with BDD and how they deal with patients who have BDD.[3] Approximately 70 percent of ASAPS members responded to the survey. Ninety-three percent (93%) of the responding members indicated that they have observed at least one of the common behaviors associate with BDD, the most frequent of which was the excessive concern with a minor or nonexistent appearance flaw. On average, plastic surgeons estimated that 2 percent of the patients seen in the initial cosmetic consultation may suffer from BDD.[4] Interestingly, this survey is consistent with the 2 percent incident rate of BBD noted in the general population. However, other studies investigating the prevalence of BDD among people who seek cosmetic surgery have indicated a higher incidence of BDD in this group than in the general population.[5] This finding indicates that we as plastic surgeons may not be recognizing BDD in some of our patients.

What occurs to BDD patients who are not diagnosed with this disorder by the plastic surgeon and undergo cosmetic surgery? According to Sarwer's survey, only 1 percent of the plastic surgeons reported a resolution of the patient's concerns. Seventeen percent reported some improvement in the patient's concern level. Thirty-nine percent indicated that the surgery solved the original problem, but the patient became focused on a different perceived defect. However, what was truly concerning was the fact that 43 percent of the plastic surgeons stated that surgery made the problem worse.[6]

Clearly, plastic surgeons need to be aware of BDD and be able to recognize this condition prior to treating patients. Most plastic surgeons believe that they can diagnose BDD in potential patients. Unfortunately, we will invariably miss the diagnosis in some of the patients presenting for consultation. When BDD patients are undiagnosed, the perceived surgical result is unpredictable, potentially leading to devastating consequences, as may be seen in the following case from my private practice.

An attractive 36-year-old professional woman came into my office in the summer of 1998 complaining of being "butchered" by whom I knew to be one of the finest plastic surgeons in Chicago. During this initial consultation, she stated that she consulted with him to potentially treat her cheeks. She felt that her cheeks were too full and lacked definition, giving her face a very round look. She wanted him to provide greater definition to her cheekbones and create a thinner face by removing some of the fat in her cheeks. He proceeded with removal of the cheek fat pads (buccal fat pads) through a well-described and accepted procedure. Subsequently, she felt that the procedure made her appear older and asymmetrical. She attempted to correct this with having cheek implants placed by another surgeon. Following placement of the cheek implants, she felt that she no longer recognized herself in the mirror anymore. She believed that the area around her eyes appeared hollow. She came to see me at that point asking for fat to be placed in her cheeks to correct the hollowness. I did not think that she needed the procedure and, even if she did, I did not believe that she was a good surgical candidate from a psychological standpoint.

She then sought another well-known plastic surgeon to undergo lifting of the cheeks using a midface lift. She believed that this procedure would make her look younger and maybe improve the sunken appearance around the eyes. After undergoing this third procedure, she remained unhappy because the surgery did not achieve what she hoped it would. She had started her quest in 1995, and by 2000 she had undergone 14 procedures on her face. She said that all of this was in an attempt to look the way she did prior to any surgical intervention.

Although I repeatedly elected not to operate on her, she continued to consult with me regarding potential corrective surgery. After several such consultations, it became apparent that she wanted to look symmetrical. I explained that no one is symmetrical, but she was convinced that, at a subconscious level, she was perceived as unattractive due to the inherent asymmetry. Yet she was as close to symmetry as the majority of attractive people. In fact, to an objective observer, she was very attractive. She focused on the perception that when she smiled, her right eye was slightly smaller than her left eye. Objectively, the difference in size was very minor and would probably be found in the majority of people. But she called this slight asymmetry a "deformity" and described herself as a life-form of a Picasso cubist sketch. She truly believed that this was the reason men did not find her attractive. She also believed that if she were able to correct this "deformity," she would be happy.

She spent her days and nights evaluating her photographs prior to surgery and those subsequent to each of her surgeries. She brought these photographs into my office. Each was labeled with typed captions and arrows describing all of the changes that took place following the various procedures. She sought the attention of a psychiatrist in order to deal with all of the stress in her life brought on by the surgeries. She was suicidal during several episodes and required hospitalization. Subsequently, she was placed on antidepressants and antipsychotic medications to enable her to function to some degree.

During the five years in which these surgeries took place, she lost her father, lost her job, endured a divorce, gained a considerable amount of weight, and, in her own words "became a social recluse," while her ex-husband remarried and created a new family. Following all of these events, she unsuccessfully attempted suicide several times. During an office visit in August 2000, I questioned her as to the source of these suicide attempts. She simply replied "it's the eye asymmetry."

I asked her if she thought she would ever be happy. She said only if she achieves perfect facial symmetry, and if that were not possible, she would probably try to commit suicide again. By March 2001, she was re-hospitalized for an attempted suicide. When I saw her again in

November 2001, she explained that the source of all of her personal and social problems lay in the first surgery that she ever had. She was on her way to New York to seek consultation with yet another plastic surgeon to inject fat back into her face.

Will she be happy with the result of his surgery, even if it is a complete success? The surgery will address the physical aspect of her facial features, not the emotional aspect. Consequently, it will not measure up to her expectations. I think the procedure will have the same pattern of emotional investment as all of the previous procedures. Her hope is that it will address all of her concerns regarding her face. Obviously, the preoccupation with the perceived asymmetry in her face is a symptom of the underlying Body Dysmorphic Disorder. As with other aspects of medicine, addressing the symptom does not treat the underlying disease.

WHERE DOES BODY DYSMORPHIC DISORDER ORIGINATE?

According to Phillips, the cause of BDD is largely unknown.[7] Multiple theories have been proposed. In the past, most theories have incorporated a psychiatric, social, or cultural basis for the disease. More recently, as with other psychiatric conditions, a biological etiology has been proposed.

There is preliminary evidence that the serotonin pathways in the brain may be involved in the etiology of BDD.[8] Serotonin is a chemical normally found in the brain. Serotonin is critical in many behavioral functions, including mood, thought process, appetite, sexual and eating behavior, and many others. It has multiple and varied roles due to different types of receptors in the brain that accept serotonin. These pathways have also been implicated in the etiology of depression and obsessive compulsive disorder.[9] Could BDD be a manifestation of these two psychiatric disorders?

Those who favor a psychological explanation suggest that BDD arises from unconscious displacement of sexual or emotional conflicts, or feelings of inferiority, guilt, or poor self-image, onto a body part. This displacement is thought to occur because the underlying problem is too threatening or difficult to be dealt with directly. The patient places his or her concerns in the more direct and manageable area of physical appearance.[10]

Some have even speculated that the body part of concern is symbolic of another, more threatening body part. Phillips gives the example of the patient who focuses on the size of his nose, whereas his true concerns revolved around the size of his penis.[11] In addition, theories incorporating the psychological basis of BDD speculate that this condition is used as a crutch for personal and professional failures in one's life.[12] It is much easier and less threatening to self-esteem to blame one's appearance than to admit lacking the social, intellectual, and emotional skills needed to function in other arenas of life.

An attractive 34-year-old woman came to my office in January 2000. She was 5'5", 120 pounds, with strawberry-blond hair and light-green eyes. Although she had lovely features and a great complexion, she did not wear any makeup. She was very conservatively dressed and sat with a slight slouch. She made very little eye contact during our conversation. She wished to consult with me regarding her breasts. She felt that she had an inadequate breast size and wished to undergo a breast augmentation. As the consultation progressed, she explained that the reason she was still single was because of her inadequate breast size. She had not been on a date in years and did not consider herself to be a desirable companion due to her small breasts. Her physical examination revealed that she was approximately a size B cup. This is hardly too small. But it was much easier to blame her physical appearance for the lack of an intimate relationship than to admit her failure in interpersonal or social skills.

Certainly, social and cultural expectations influence our perceptions of ourselves. The way in which we are treated as children affects how we perceive ourselves as adults. My patient described earlier who attempted suicide had a younger sister who was always described by the family as the "pretty one," whereas my patient was described as the "smart one." She never saw herself as being as attractive as her younger sister.

The media constantly reminds us of the importance of looking our best. We are encouraged to address our imperfections. Many advertisements for cosmetic procedures promote self-doubt and the pursuit of perfection. If someone has a low self-esteem from childhood events or from an abusive personal relationship, he or she will be more vulnerable to these influences. When we constantly measure ourselves against others who are more attractive, we are certain to become critical of ourselves. It is only natural to do so. However, it is unhealthy to focus on every flaw and overlook any positive attributes.

As with other psychiatric disorders, most likely the origin of BDD is multifactorial. There are probably neurological, biological, psychological, and social influences. If an individual has the biological predisposition, then the psychological or social impacts may trigger BDD. In order for BDD to be diagnosed, it must be ascertained that the physical defect is nonexistent or slight. The following are the questions that Phillips suggests asking to help identify the possible presence of BDD:[13]

1. Are you overly concerned about the appearance of some part(s) of your body which you consider unattractive?
2. If yes, do these concerns preoccupy your thoughts?
3. Do you wish you could spend less time thinking about your appearance flaw?
4. Do you spend at least one hour per day thinking about your appearance flaw?
5. Have your appearance concerns affected your life?
6. Are there things you avoid because of your appearance?
7. Have your appearance concerns caused you a lot of distress or emotional pain?

If the answer is yes to some of these questions, we need to consider the possibility that BDD may be the underlying causative factor. In these cases, it is important to recognize that psychiatric treatment is available and may be of benefit.

5

Plastic Surgery and Adolescents

As we discuss the impact of plastic surgery on self-esteem, a question arises regarding the role of plastic surgery in the lives of children and adolescents. According to surveys conducted by the American Society of Plastic Surgeons (ASPS), children between the ages of 13 to 19 years of age make up approximately 2 percent of the cosmetic surgery patients in the United States.[1] Is it a good idea to consider cosmetic surgery in children and adolescents? When should we surgically intervene in a child's life for the purpose of improving his or her appearance? There is no doubt that reconstructive surgery such as the repair of cleft lip or other congenital conditions is more than appropriate and greatly benefits the child. The controversial procedures include the purely elective cosmetic ones being performed in healthy children or adolescents who do not have any congenital or acquired physical defects. Which cosmetic procedures are reasonable to consider in children or adolescents? Which cosmetic procedures should be avoided in this group?

The first question that we need to answer is, why are children or adolescents seeking elective surgery? Usually, they seek cosmetic surgery in an effort to "fit in." The media has greatly emphasized the role of cosmetic surgery in adolescents. This has gone to the extent of publicizing that breast augmentation procedures are now requested as high school graduation gifts. As children and adolescents become more aware of the cosmetic procedures that can be performed, and as they witness young celebrities undergoing these procedures, it is only natural that they begin considering surgery for what they perceive to be their own flaws.

Which cosmetic surgery procedures may be considered appropriate for adolescents? In general, conditions that present during a young age and are known not to change with normal growth patterns are reasonable to address in adolescents, assuming that the adolescent is an appropriate candidate. How do we determine if adolescents who are not even legally permitted to authorize written consent are appropriate surgical candidates? They must be evaluated in the same manner as adult patients. Adolescents must demonstrate an ability to understand the procedure, have appropriate coping skills for the recovery, have realistic expectations for the outcome, confirm that the procedure is their own idea and not for the intention of pleasing someone else, convey that the condition for which they are seeking treatment has troubled them on a regular basis and is not simply a seldom concern, and clearly establish that their perception of the physical flaw is consistent with what is actually present on a physical exam. Once these criteria are met, the cosmetic surgery procedures that may be appropriate for adolescents include the following:

- *Otoplasty (ear setback surgery)* is appropriate in children as young as five years of age. By then, the cartilage in the ears is well developed and more likely to maintain the new shape into which it is molded. Often, we perform this procedure before the child starts school in an effort to prevent any psychological trauma arising from other children's ridicule. As such, an otoplasty may be performed on anyone over five years of age and is tolerated quite well by this patient population.

- *Rhinoplasty* may be considered in adolescents once the face has completed growth. Usually, facial features reach adult proportions after the completion of puberty. As such, it is safe to consider rhinoplasty in girls after 14 or 15 years of age and in boys after 15 or 16 years of age. This procedure can have a dramatic positive effect on adolescents during those difficult years when they are experiencing and questioning many of their physical changes.

- *Breast reduction* is a good procedure for adolescent girls who have completed puberty, have significantly enlarged breasts, and have physical symptoms thought to be related to the enlarged breasts (see Chapter 18). Most girls complete puberty by 15 years of age, at which time the extent of breast growth is reasonably well established. Whenever possible, it is best to ensure that the breast growth has stopped and the breast size has remained stable for at least one year. It is also important for anyone considering a reduction mammaplasty to be at a stable body weight. The individual's weight has an impact not only on their original breast size, but also on the breast size that would be most appropriate to achieve with surgery. If the patient loses a great deal of weight after a breast reduction, the breast size that may have seemed appropriate immediately following surgery may then appear too small.

- *Breast asymmetry* is usually noted at a very young age. Although all women have some degree of breast asymmetry, there are situations in which the asymmetry is more than what is considered normal. Under these circumstances, usually one breast has developed completely and the other is minimally developed or not developed at all. A significant degree of asymmetry will not drastically improve on its own. It usually presents considerable psychological stress for most adolescent girls. Some cases may be addressed simply with different size implants to achieve greater symmetry. Some patients may require a breast reduction with a breast lift and a small implant for the larger breast and simply a larger implant for the smaller breast. Patients often wonder why an implant is needed for the larger of the two breasts. The reason is that an implanted breast looks quite different from a breast without an implant. An implanted breast will have fullness along the upper pole, whereas a breast without an implant usually lacks this fullness. If the goal is to achieve better symmetry, then both breasts usually require an implant.

- *Gynecomastia* presents a significant psychological stress for most young boys. They are afraid to remove their shirts in public due to fear of being ridiculed. Fortunately, most cases of gynecomastia resolve on their own by the time the child has completed puberty. The incidence drops to less than 10 percent in boys over 17 years of age and begins to rise again after middle age. The majority of the time, gynecomastia occurs without a known cause and is a normal finding. However at any age, it can be associated with an underlying disease or the use of medications or recreational drugs and warrants evaluation by a qualified physician (see Chapter 21).

The two most controversial procedures in adolescents are liposuction and breast augmentation. Liposuction should never be used for weight management at any age. It is indicated as a contouring tool for areas that do not respond to diet and exercise. Adolescents experience significant changes in their bodies due to normal growth. It is difficult to predict how these changes will mature over time. Intervening with liposuction may prove to be unnecessary once the adolescent has fully developed.

Furthermore, providing liposuction as an option for an adolescent may have significant psychological ramifications in the future. All adolescents need to learn how to manage their weight with diet and exercise. If they undergo liposuction at an impressionable age and see it as a quick alternative to more traditional ways of weight management, they may not strive to develop the habits needed to maintain a healthy weight later in life. Finally, eating disorders often manifest during adolescence and liposuction may be misused.

As with liposuction, breast augmentation should be avoided in adolescents. In 2004, ASPS took an official stand against breast augmentation in women under 18 years of age. The Food and Drug Administration (FDA) approves saline breast implants for women 18 years of age or older and silicone breast implants for women 22 years of age or older. However, it is legal for physicians to perform breast augmentation on women under 18 years of age under what is considered an off-label use.

There are several reasons to avoid breast augmentations in adolescent girls. Some girls experience changes in the size of their breasts during later adolescent years, and may have sufficient breast growth to eliminate the desire for breast enlargement. Unlike breast reductions, breast augmentations are purely cosmetic and have more significant future implications. Breast implants are not considered lifetime devices and require additional surgery throughout the individual's life. Undergoing breast augmentation at a young age dictates a higher number of breast implant revisions and replacements over time. An adolescent may not fully appreciate the significance of the risks and costs associated with numerous surgeries.

6

Choosing a Plastic Surgeon

How do you decide who will perform your surgery? After all, you are entrusting this surgeon with your face or your body. You are expecting this surgeon to have a great understanding of what you wish to achieve. You are expecting this surgeon to have the ability to unite surgical skill with an artistic sense that mirrors your sense of aesthetics.

Where do you find such a surgeon? You need to start with a list of good candidates. With the great deal of advertising that is currently used by many physicians, it is difficult for a patient to identify who is truly qualified. Unfortunately, some physicians may advertise in a manner that can be quite misleading. The following are some guidelines for creating your list of candidates.

1. Obtain plastic surgeons' names from your family doctor or gynecologist. They see patients who have had plastic surgery with favorable and unfavorable results and would have valuable recommendations of doctors' names. In rare cases, patients have told me that their primary care physician does not "believe in" plastic surgery. Under these circumstances, it is best to consider other sources of referrals.

2. Check with your friends who have undergone the procedure that you are considering. These friends can be a very valuable source of information. It is important to obtain more than one doctor's name, since individual experiences vary. You may have a very different outcome from that of your friend who underwent surgery by the same surgeon. All surgeons will have some great results, and all surgeons will have some complications.

3. If you have friends who work in surgical centers or hospitals where plastic surgery is performed, they can be a great source

of information. They are typically exposed to plastic surgeons or to nurses and anesthesiologists working with plastic surgeons. They can usually provide names of qualified plastic surgeons.

4. Check with your hairdresser, aesthetician, or makeup artist. They see many women who have undergone face lifts and can usually provide good references. Their input is very valuable, especially if they have multiple clients who underwent surgery by the same surgeon.

5. The other sources of obtaining plastic surgeons names include the American Society of Plastic Surgeons (ASPS) and the American Society for Aesthetic Plastic Surgery (ASAPS). ASPS is the largest organization of plastic surgeons in the United States. In order to become a member of ASPS, the plastic surgeon must have completed a full residency in plastic surgery and must be certified by the American Board of Plastic Surgery. In order to become a member of ASAPS, the plastic surgeon must demonstrate that he or she has performed a significant number of aesthetic (cosmetic) procedures.

Once you have compiled a list of candidates, then you need to investigate each surgeon's credentials and specialty by addressing the following:

1. *Training*: All plastic surgeons must complete 6 to 10 years of surgical training following graduation from medical school. This begins with prerequisite training in a qualified field of surgery, such as general surgery, otolaryngology, or oral surgery. This is then followed by surgical training, specifically in an accredited plastic surgery training program. These programs consist of an additional two to three years of very intense training in all aspects of reconstructive and cosmetic plastic surgery. Some plastic surgeons continue their education and obtain additional training in a more specific field of plastic surgery, such as craniofacial surgery, breast surgery, or hand surgery.

2. *Board certification*: Over the past decade, patients have been advised to seek surgeons who are "board-certified." Unfortunately, that term has been misused. More recently, "boards" have been created to suggest that physicians have special training in a field of plastic surgery. It is important to know the exact name of the board in which your surgeon has been granted certification. Be sure that it is a board recognized by the American Board of Medical Specialties (ABMS). Plastic surgeons completing proper

training are eligible to obtain certification by the American Board of Plastic Surgery. The certification process by the American Board of Plastic Surgery is very rigorous. It requires both written and oral examinations. In addition, it requires demonstration of surgical competence and ethics. This is accomplished by a thorough review of all surgeries performed and their outcomes during the surgeon's first two years in practice. Currently, the American Board of Plastic Surgery issues certificates that are effective for only 10 years. Renewal of the board certificate requires a lengthy process that begins with the plastic surgeon submitting a six-month case list of surgeries performed and their outcomes. Based on the type of procedures performed, the surgeon must complete a written examination specific to his or her practice in plastic surgery. This rigorous procedure ensures that the board-certified plastic surgeon is current in the specific field of plastic surgery practiced. The American Board of Medical Specialties provides a listing of all of the legitimate boards in medicine. Be cautious and thoroughly research surgeons claiming that they have board certification by a board not recognized by the American Board of Medical Specialties.

3. *Hospital privileges*: All plastic surgeons should have hospital privileges, even if they perform surgery in an accredited office or surgical center. The hospital privileges dictate which procedures the surgeon is allowed to perform based on his or her credentials. This list is annually reviewed and approved by the chairman and credentialing committee of the hospital. Furthermore, having hospital privileges allows the surgeon to admit patients should there be a complication following surgery that necessitates hospitalization.

4. *Malpractice coverage*: All practicing plastic surgeons should carry malpractice insurance. Proof of insurance is required by all hospitals and surgical centers before granting surgical privileges to the surgeon. Lack of malpractice coverage warrants further investigation. It is unlikely that the plastic surgeon does not have insurance because he or she chooses not to carry a policy. More likely, it is because he or she is unable to obtain malpractice coverage due to previous malpractice claims or judgments.

5. *State medical board*: Each state has a governing board that grants physicians medical licenses to practice medicine. It does not dictate which type of medical specialty the physician can practice and is unrelated to the boards that specify a physician's specialty (e.g., American Board of Plastic Surgery, American Board of

Otolaryngology, American Board of Dermatology, etc.). The state medical board can provide valuable information regarding a physician, including: medical education and surgical training; the number of malpractice claims; and the status of the physician's license. A history of malpractice claims does not by itself suggest that the surgeon is not competent. If the surgeon has a high number of medical malpractice claims or a history of having his or her license revoked for any period of time, it indicates more serious competence issues.

6. *Subspecialty*: Plastic surgery includes both reconstructive and cosmetic procedures. The reconstructive procedures are those that repair an acquired or congenital deformity (e.g., facial injuries following automobile accidents, cleft lip and palate in children, and breast reconstruction following breast cancer treatment). The cosmetic procedures are elective procedures intended to improve one's appearance (e.g., face lift, breast augmentation, and liposuction). All well-established plastic surgeons have procedures that they perform more frequently than others. First, find out if the plastic surgeon performs mainly reconstructive or cosmetic procedures. Second, find out which procedures the surgeon performs regularly. In essence, you are trying to determine the surgeon's subspecialty. Your procedure of interest should be included in that list. Finally, find out if your plastic surgeon is a member of the ASAPS. This is a good indication that the surgeon performs a significant number of cosmetic procedures.

Once you have consolidated your list, then it is to your benefit to meet with two or three plastic surgeons in order to choose one who meets your needs. During the consultation, you should consider the following:

1. You should feel comfortable. You need to feel at ease with the person you are entrusting with your face or body. You should feel that the surgeon understands you and understands the changes that you wish to create.

2. You should be given a reasonable amount of time with the surgeon. If the practice "consultant" or "patient coordinator" meets with you, discusses the procedure and recovery, but the surgeon drops in for only a few minutes, then you should realize that you will have very little contact with your surgeon in that type of practice.

3. All of your questions should be taken seriously and answered thoroughly.

4. Be very cautious of surgeons who suggest many more procedures than you were initially considering. For example, if you present to a surgeon desiring treatment of your upper eyelids and he or she suggests treating the lower eyelids at the same time, it is within reason. However, if you present desiring your eyes to be treated and then find that the surgeon is also recommending a face lift and neck lift with possible chin implant, etc., be careful and obtain another opinion.

5. Your surgeon's first goal should be your safety. If you find that your surgeon encourages you to undergo procedures without a thorough evaluation of your medical history or without obtaining medical clearance from your internist when indicated, you need to be cautious. If you plan to have several procedures involving different areas of the body (e.g., face lift, breast lift, breast augmentation, and tummy tuck), and your surgeon encourages you to undergo all of these at the same time, you have to question his or her judgment. Any procedure that requires many hours of general anesthesia places you at high risk. Furthermore, the longer you are under general anesthesia, the longer your recovery will be.

6. You should also have the sense that should there be a complication, this person will be there to carry you through to a full recovery. This can sometimes be predicted by the amount of attention you receive from the surgeon before your surgery.

7. Finally, you should like and respect your surgeon and believe that these feelings are mutual.

7

Preparing for Your Surgery

You have thought about your plastic surgery for weeks, months, or maybe even years. You went to seek the advice of several reputable board-certified plastic surgeons and selected the one you feel is best suited for your needs. You have set the date and rearranged your work schedule and your family's schedule around this date. You have come to terms with why you want this done. You accept the risks, the recovery, the costs, and the uncertainty. You have spoken to your best friend and confidant about your surgery for moral support. Now, how do you prepare?

Like most patients, your friends have probably given you solicited and unsolicited advice regarding what you should and should not do. With so much information from friends who have had the same procedure and the worldwide web chat rooms of patients more than willing to share their experience, how do you filter out what pertains to you? Are there medications that help you have less swelling after surgery? Is Arnica good or bad? Should you take Arnica before or after surgery? What is Arnica? Should you lose weight before liposuction? Should you stop taking birth control pills before a breast augmentation? What can you do to decrease bruising after surgery? Are herbal supplements good to take prior to your procedure? Are herbal supplements dangerous to take prior to your procedure? Do you need to see your internist or family doctor before plastic surgery? Where do you begin?

This chapter is intended to give patients basic recommendations for preparing for surgery so as to optimize their recovery and potential outcome. These recommendations are designed to apply to the average patient. Should your health history indicate, there may be additional recommendations provided by your surgeon, which should be followed to increase the safety of your surgery.

The month prior to plastic surgery is an important time in your life. You may view it as the preparation phase. You can take this time to do everything you can to optimize your surgery and your recovery. Not only should you be mentally prepared, but you should be physically prepared. The surgery may be viewed as a test of your physical and mental health. Just like any other test in life, the more prepared you are, the better you will do.

THE MONTH PRIOR TO YOUR SURGERY

Do You Smoke?

If so, do you know that your healing will be compromised? Nicotine in any form (cigarettes, gum, chewing tobacco, transdermal patches) will decrease the blood supply to the skin. This may have serious consequences in procedures in which lifting of the skin is necessary, such as face lifts, tummy tucks, breast lifts or reductions, and thigh and buttock lifts. Many plastic surgeons will not perform these procedures on smokers. In these patients, the skin will not have an adequate blood supply and may slough, leading to non-healing wounds or terrible scarring.

Eliminating nicotine from your system will allow you to heal better, even for procedures in which skin is not lifted. The length of time one should be nicotine-free depends upon the type of procedure that is planned as well as the amount of nicotine they use on a daily basis. Someone who smokes two to three cigarettes per day is different from someone who smokes two packs of cigarettes per day. It is best to check with your surgeon regarding their recommendations for your particular procedure based on your own smoking history.

Do You Drink Alcohol on a Daily Basis?

Alcohol is processed by the liver, which is the organ responsible for helping our blood clot normally. Patients who drink large amounts of alcohol daily may not clot as well as needed for most delicate plastic surgery procedures. Alcohol has two possible side effects during surgery and during recovery. It can increase bleeding during surgery, leading to a greater risk of complications such as hematoma (collection of blood under the skin); or, to a lesser extent, it may lead to greater bruising. Also, the extent of bleeding may make surgery more difficult to perform, resulting in a longer procedure. This necessitates longer exposure to general anesthesia, which increases the number of risks and potential complications. Furthermore, if patients are able to decrease their alcohol intake prior to surgery, they will have an easier time not drinking after surgery, when they need to take narcotics for pain management. If they are also drinking alcohol along with pain medication, they may place themselves at serious health risks.

Do You Take Herbal Supplements or High-Dose Vitamins?

There is a new trend that we see in many patients. During a consultation, it is not unusual for a patient to report that she is taking two to three herbs and multiple high-dose vitamins, in addition to a variety of antioxidants and anti-inflammatory drugs. Many patients like to take herbs because they are "natural," and consequently, patients view them as being safe. However, patients should keep in mind that many prescribed drugs have their origin in naturally occurring substances.

Unfortunately, many herbal supplements are not well studied. Because they are herbs and considered natural, many have not been thoroughly evaluated by the FDA. They could have many risks that are currently unknown. The herbal supplements that have been studied, such as glucosamine and chondroitin sulfate, have been found to have some properties similar to blood thinners. It would be unheard of to perform an elective plastic surgery on a patient taking a blood thinner; yet patients taking glucosamine and chondroitin sulfate are presenting for elective plastic surgery on a regular basis. Furthermore, patients will receive many medications during anesthesia, and we do not know how these herbs will interact with the anesthetic drugs.

In addition to herbs, vitamin E has also been shown to increase bleeding, and as such should be discontinued prior to surgery. Patients are advised to stop taking herbs, vitamin E, aspirin, antioxidants, and anti-inflammatory medications during the month prior to surgery. Often, patients ingest powdered "health drinks" or "energy bars" that are intended to boost energy levels, improve complexion, strengthen nail and hair growth, etc. The ingredients in these drinks must be evaluated, as they often contain high levels of antioxidants, which will contribute to bleeding. A list of the herbs, vitamins, and medications to avoid is found in the Appendix.

Patients often ask about the benefits of Arnica (Arnica Montana) in plastic surgery. Arnica is an herb found in Scandinavia, southern Europe, southern Russia, and central Asia.[1] It is believed to reduce inflammation and pain. The indications and usage of Arnica approved by Commission E are: fever, cough, bronchitis, rheumatism, and inflammation of the skin.[2] Unproven indications include swelling and bruising.[3] Since these are unproven, plastic surgeons may be reluctant to routinely recommend Arnica either before or after surgery.

Are You Planning a Vacation in a Sunny Location?

It is important to avoid significant sun exposure, since a suntan along the area undergoing surgery may lead to uneven pigmentation during recovery. Avoiding sun exposure is particularly important in facial plastic surgery, and is crucial when undergoing laser resurfacing or other laser procedures. In terms of laser procedures to soften wrinkles, remove hair, reduce discoloration (brown or red), a tan often necessitates postponing the procedure, since the risks of uneven pigmentation (either loss of pigment or excessive pigment) or even burning the skin are very high. In terms of body surgery, a significant sunburn may necessitate postponing surgery due to the extent of inflammation in the area.

Does Your Weight Fluctuate Significantly?

It is important not to have a significant weight loss or weight gain prior to surgery. The best time to have surgery is when you are at a stable and safe weight. You do not want to be at your heaviest or struggle to be at your lowest weight. This is true for facial and body surgery. Excessive dieting just prior to or immediately following surgery may compromise the nutritional needs necessary for healing during recovery. Furthermore, crash dieting prior to surgery may lead to a rebound effect afterwards, causing patients to gain weight. Excessive weight gain after surgery will compromise the cosmetic result of both facial and body surgery. Patients should try to adopt a healthy diet and exercise regimen during the month prior to surgery and continue this afterwards in order to further enhance their results.

Surgeons frequently use the term "the stress of surgery" to describe how the patient physically handles the procedure. Surgery is a stress to your system. Ideally, the preoperative exercise regimen should incorporate walking or another form of aerobic exercise to improve your stamina, enhance your body's ability to handle the stress of surgery, and decrease the potential of blood clots forming in the legs and making their way to the lungs at the time of surgery. Many patients think that the only risk of a blood clot forming in the legs occurs during surgery. That is not the case. Only some of the clinically significant blood clots form during surgery. Most surgeons take the necessary precautions to decrease the risk of blood clots forming in the legs during surgery. However, surgeons cannot control the risk of these forming prior to surgery. If patients live a sedentary lifestyle, or if they are overweight, or if they have recently been on a lengthy airplane flight, the blood clot may form in the leg before the date of their surgery. Many of these blood clots are not symptomatic, and the body dissolves them without our awareness that they even existed. However, some of these blood clots are not dissolved by the body, only to become dislodged during surgery, leading to severe complications.

The timing of exercise after surgery depends upon the procedure performed. In general, patients are encouraged to walk as tolerated immediately after their procedure to further decrease risks. More aggressive exercise may be resumed after appropriate healing and evaluation by the surgeon.

Are You Having Facial Rejuvenation Surgery Such as a Face Lift, Eyelid Lift, or Laser Resurfacing?

This requires optimizing your skin tone to enhance healing. Ideally, the patient would adopt a regimen of skin care such as a series of micro-dermabrasion treatments or gentle exfoliating peels during the month prior to the facial surgery. If necessary, these may be further combined with a home care regimen consisting of retinoids, glycolic acids, or Tazorac creams. This type of preparation may improve the skin's ability to create new collagen during the healing phase after surgery.

Are You Having a Breast Augmentation, Breast Lift, or Breast Reduction?

Most women will notice a fluctuation in their weight and breast size during different points of their menstrual cycle. Usually, these fluctuations are relatively minor. However, patients taking oral contraceptives may experience greater fluctuations in weight and breast size during the use of these medications. The extent of these changes depends upon the type of oral contraceptive used and the patient's unique response. If you have experienced a noticeable increase in your breast size with the use of your current oral contraceptive, then you should discontinue its use at least one to two months prior to breast surgery and use another form of birth control during that period. This will allow your breasts to go back to their natural state, enabling a more accurate choice for either breast augmentation or reduction. If the oral contraceptive does not have much impact on breast size, there is less of a need to discontinue its use. Some surgeons advise patients to discontinue all oral contraceptives prior to surgery, since they increase the risk of blood clots.

As part of your preoperative assessment, you may need to undergo a bilateral mammogram. If you are age 35 to 40 and have never had a mammogram, or over the age of 40 and have not had a mammogram within the preceeding year, you need a mammogram. Also, if you have had an abnormal mammogram, an abnormal breast exam, or a family history of breast disease, you need a mammogram prior to your surgery.

Are You Over 50 Years of Age, or Do You Have Any Preexisting Medical Conditions?

If so, it is important to meet with your internist to receive medical clearance prior to your surgery. This visit usually includes a thorough physical and blood tests and, in some cases, may include studies such as an EKG (heart evaluation) and a chest X-ray. It ensures that you do not have additional risks that will compromise your health during the surgery or the recovery period. Meeting with your internist early enough allows the time for proper workup of any abnormal findings and prevents unnecessary postponing of your surgery.

THE WEEK PRIOR TO SURGERY

- Drink an average of eight glasses of water per day to ensure that your body is well hydrated prior to your surgery.
- Have all of your prescriptions filled so they will be home upon your return from surgery.
- If you are having a face lift or a brow lift and you color your hair, do so at least one week prior to surgery, as you will not be able to color it for approximately four weeks after surgery.
- Be sure to immediately inform your surgeon if you develop a cold sore, fever blister, cold or flu-like symptoms, or a fever. These may require additional precautions or postponing your procedure.
- Obtain and prepare items that you will need during your recovery, such as:
  - Light, healthy foods that do not require much preparation.
  - Favorite fruit juices, Gatorade, and water, since you will need to stay well hydrated after surgery.
  - Magazines, books, and movies to help you manage your time during the recovery period.
  - Comfortable, loose clothing that buttons in the front, to minimize pulling anything over your head or raising your arms.
  - Comfortable slippers, as you will spend much of your time lounging.

o Multiple pillows (three to four), as you may need to sleep in several different positions in order to find a comfortable one.

o Stool softeners, since the pain medications prescribed and lack of exercise immediately after surgery often lead to constipation. These may include glycerin suppositories as well as oral stool softeners. If you know that you are prone to constipation, or if the surgery requires prolonged use of pain medication, it is best to be proactive and begin taking stool softeners the day after surgery.

o If you are having a breast procedure, ask your surgeon about the type of bra you will need during the first two to four weeks following your surgery, and obtain at least two of these.

o If you are having liposuction, have several old towels or blankets available to cover your couch or bed should there be any drainage from the incisions during the first couple of days after surgery.

o If you are having a facial procedure:

1. Obtain camouflage makeup and learn how to apply it.
2. Obtain two to three ice packs to help decrease bruising after surgery (some find it helpful to use bags of frozen peas).
3. Obtain an ointment such as Aquaphor to apply along exposed surgical incisions to help them remain moist, feel more comfortable, and heal well.
4. Have cotton swabs available to use in cleaning the wounds and applying ointment.

THE DAY PRIOR TO SURGERY

- Eat a light healthy diet. Avoid spicy foods, as these tend to cause water retention.

- In the evening prior to going to sleep, wash the area that will undergo surgery with a medicated antimicrobial soap such as Hibiclens.

- Avoid staying up late. If you are very anxious and think that you will be unable to sleep the night prior to your surgery, discuss with your surgeon the possibility of taking a sleeping pill to help you.

THE MORNING OF SURGERY

- Shower and wash your hair, as you may not be able to do this immediately after surgery. Avoid creams, antiperspirants, hair-styling products, makeup, perfumes, contact lenses, and jewelry.

- Wash the area that will undergo surgery with the medicated soap once again.
- Have a responsible adult drive you to the center where surgery will be performed, and arrange for them to pick you up after surgery. You should not drive by yourself or be alone with an unfamiliar driver.

Surgical Approaches to Facial Rejuvenation and Enhancement

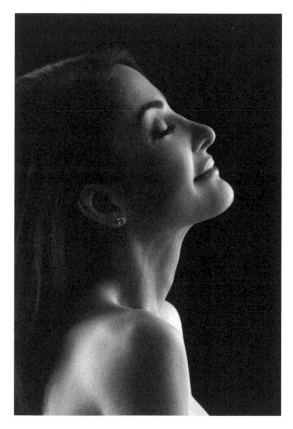

Stuart Rogers Photography

8

Face Lift (Rhytidectomy)

WHAT IS A FACE LIFT, AND WHAT DOES IT ACCOMPLISH?

- A face lift tightens the lax tissues of the cheeks, jowls, and neck (Fig. 8.1).
- A face lift is not the procedure of choice to treat prominent naso-labial folds (the depressions extending from the side of the nose down to the mouth).
- It is more effective for the lower face and neck than for the upper face.
- It restores the jaw line definition and neck profile.
- The extent of the face lift surgery needs to be individualized for each patient, depending on the degree of tissue sagging.
- A face lift can be performed alone or along with other procedures, such as a brow lift, neck liposuction, eyelid surgery, or nasal surgery.

HOW IS A FACE LIFT PERFORMED?

- The earliest face lifts were done by simply excising some skin from the area in front of the ear and closing the two edges of tissue together. This gave the cheek a lifted and improved appearance, but the results were short-lived. In addition, the scars from this type of procedure tended to widen, since all of the tension resulting from the skin closure was placed on the skin.
- As the understanding of anatomy and surgical principles developed, the modern techniques of face lifting were introduced.

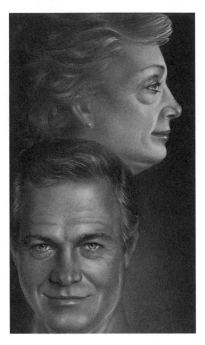

Figure 8.1. A face lift can improve the deep cheek folds, the jowls, and the loose, sagging skin around the neck that result from aging. (Courtesy American Society of Plastic Surgeons.)

- The skin incision usually begins behind the hairline at the level of the temples, follows the natural crease in front of the ear (or is placed inside the ear), curves behind the earlobe into the crease behind the ear, and follows the hairline into the posterior scalp. There may also be a small incision in the neck just beneath the chin to access the neck (Fig. 8.2).
- We now understand that it is the layer of connective tissue and attached muscles just beneath the surface of the skin that contribute greatly to facial laxity over time. This structure is called the SMAS.
- This abbreviation SMAS stands for *Superficial Musculo Aponeurotic System.*
  - *Superficial:* Refers to the location of this structure since it is just beneath the fatty layer of the skin.
  - *Musculo:* Refers to the presence of a thin muscle sheet under the fatty layer of the skin. In the neck, this is known as the *platysma muscle.* The platysma extends from the lower aspect of the neck to the jawline.

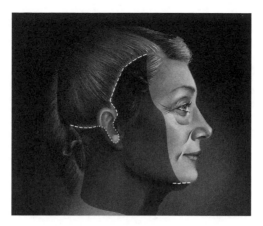

Figure 8.2. Incisions usually begin behind the hairline at the level of the temples, follow the natural skin line in front of the ear, curve behind the earlobe into the crease behind the ear, and into or along the lower scalp. (Courtesy American Society of Plastic Surgeons.)

It then extends into the cheeks, not as a muscle but as a connective tissue layer known as the *aponeurosis*.

- The SMAS forms a system that allows the deep muscles of facial expression to transmit forces to the overlying skin. These are the muscles that are responsible for facial movement (for example, smiling, frowning, etc.). When the deeper muscles of facial expression contract, the muscle fibers pull on the SMAS, which in turn pulls on the skin. The skin itself is a very elastic structure and will simply contour to the underlying structures and vectors of pull.
- As we continuously use our muscles of facial expression over the course of years, the SMAS stretches and loosens and eventually sags, causing the overlying facial skin to sag as well.

- Modern face lifting involves tightening the SMAS layer beneath the surface of the skin in addition to tightening the skin. By placing most or all of the tension on the SMAS layer, we avoid a stretched and mask-like appearance to the skin itself. This results in a much more natural result and less of a "surgical look." It also prevents tension on the incisions, allowing the scars to heal well.
- There are three basic ways to tighten the SMAS.

  - The easiest and least risky is to tighten the SMAS on its surface by sewing parts of it together.
  - The second way is to surgically cut a wedge out of the SMAS and tighten the SMAS by sewing the two edges together.

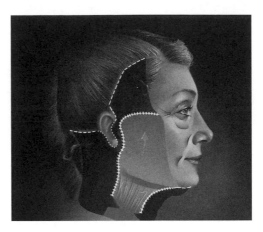

Figure 8.3. The facial and neck skin may be separated from the underlying muscle; fat may be trimmed or suctioned, and the underlying muscle may be tightened. (Courtesy American Society of Plastic Surgeons.)

- o The third technique, an extension of the second, is technically more demanding. It involves surgically cutting into the SMAS and releasing it from the underlying structures. The extra and loose SMAS tissue is then cut away, and the remaining SMAS is anchored in its new uplifted position (Fig. 8.3). Of the three techniques, this technique carries the greatest risk of facial nerve damage, since the facial nerve runs under the SMAS. Elevation of the SMAS makes various branches of the facial nerve vulnerable.

- The specific technique used depends on what the patient and surgeon are trying to accomplish, the type of tissue the patient has, and the surgical skill and comfort of the surgeon.

- In addition to tightening the SMAS and overlying skin, completion of the face lift requires addressing the neck either with liposuction alone, or liposuction in conjunction with tightening of the platysma muscle to improve the neck contour (Fig. 8.4).

- After tightening the SMAS, the skin is lifted into its new position, the excess skin is trimmed, and the incisions are closed with very fine sutures (Figs. 8.4, 8.5). Most plastic surgeons will use sutures that do not need to be removed, but dissolve on their own within approximately one week after surgery.

WHERE ARE THE INCISIONS PLACED?

- This is another important aspect of the final results of a face lift. The placement of the incision must preserve the hair tuft

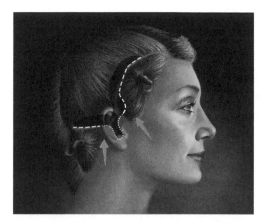

Figure 8.4. After the deep tissues are tightened, the excess skin is pulled up and back, trimmed, and sutured into place. (Courtesy American Society of Plastic Surgeons.)

located in front of the upper aspect of the ear. If this hair tuft is shifted, reduced, or removed, it will give a very obvious surgical appearance to the face and also makes hairstyling very difficult for the patient. The placement of the incision must also preserve the hairline behind the ear, as shifting this may also have similar consequences.

- The incision starts either in the natural skin crease where the ear meets the face, or just inside the ear. Many plastic surgeons

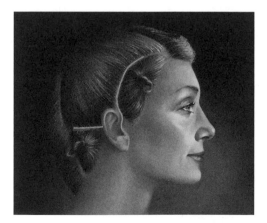

Figure 8.5. Most of the scars will be hidden within your hair and in the normal creases of your skin. (Courtesy American Society of Plastic Surgeons.)

prefer to place the incision inside the ear whenever possible, as this minimizes its visibility. Superiorly, the incision is then carried into the hair-bearing scalp toward the temple, and inferiorly, it curves around the earlobe and extends behind the ear and into the hair-bearing part of the scalp. There is often one small incision beneath the chin, either for liposuction of the neck (3–5 mm) or for liposuction and muscle tightening of the neck (2–2.5 cm).

HOW LONG IS THE RECOVERY PERIOD FOLLOWING A FACE LIFT?

- The recovery time is approximately two weeks. Most of the bruising and swelling can be covered up with makeup after 7–10 days. However, we advise most patients to give themselves a period of two weeks for recovery.

DOES A FACE LIFT HURT?

- Although everyone is different, most patients state that there is very little pain after a face lift.
- However, many patients experience discomfort the first night from the dressing wrapped around the face and neck. This dressing is removed the next morning after surgery, and a different garment is worn for the first week after surgery.
- Although pain medication is prescribed, most patients do not need to be medicated beyond the first few days after surgery. During the initial period, the majority of the discomfort is due to a feeling of tightness in the jawline and neck regions, as well as pain along the incisions inside and around the ears. The tightness relaxes over time, and the pain dissipates over the first few days following surgery.

ARE THERE ANY SCARS?

- There are scars, but these run in the natural creases of the skin, inside the ear, and in the hairline.
- Usually the scars cannot be easily seen.
- Rarely, patients may experience thickening of the face lift scars.

WHAT KIND OF ANESTHESIA IS RECOMMENDED DURING A FACE LIFT?

- Twilight anesthesia (local anesthesia with sedation) or general anesthesia is recommended during a face lift. More extensive face lift procedures are usually performed under general anesthesia.

WHERE SHOULD A FACE LIFT BE PERFORMED?

- A face lift may be performed in a hospital, an outpatient surgical center, or an appropriately accredited office operating room.
- If a doctor elects to perform the procedure in the office, the patient must be certain that the office operating room is accredited by one of the state's accreditation associations. Otherwise, the safety of the operating room is not as reliable.

WHAT CAN I EXPECT AFTER FACE LIFT SURGERY?

- When you awaken in the recovery room following your face lift, you will have a dressing wrapped around your neck, cheeks, and scalp, leaving your eyes, nose, and mouth exposed. This dressing usually consists of gauze and an elastic wrap. It is required to remain in place overnight in order to provide slight compression over your face and reduce the amount of bruising and swelling that you will experience. However, it is important that the dressing not be too tight, as it can compromise the blood supply to the skin.
- The swelling and bruising actually worsen during the first few days following surgery. Your maximum swelling and bruising occur not immediately after the face lift, but are usually experienced approximately 48 hours following surgery. Subsequently, the swelling begins to stabilize and diminish. The bruising begins to turn from a dark red to a purple color. Finally, the bruises begin to turn yellow as they fade. They may make their way down onto the neck. Some surgeons prefer the use of drains to decrease the amount of bruising and swelling after surgery. These drains are typically removed the next morning after surgery, when the initial bandages are removed.
- Immediately after surgery, you can expect to be quite swollen along the cheeks, in front of the ears, and on the sides of the neck. You will also feel numb in these areas. The swelling will improve

significantly during the first two weeks, and the numbness will improve over 2–12 months.

- In the first 24–48 hours, you may use cold compresses over the jaw and neck for 20–30 minutes every hour. This may help reduce some of the swelling and bruising. After the first 72 hours, warm compresses may be used to help improve the bruising.

- Once the initial swelling has resolved, it is normal to have some residual fullness or a feeling of hardness in front of the ears and across the neck. This is a natural consequence of the healing and will soften over a period of 2–6 months.

- You may experience minor irregularities along the surface of the skin immediately after surgery. These are usually due to swelling and resolve over the first few weeks after surgery as the swelling decreases.

HOW DO I CARE FOR MYSELF AFTER THE FACE LIFT SURGERY?

- After removing the initial dressing, many surgeons place the patient in an elastic facial wrap that drapes beneath the chin and over the ears. This face garment is usually worn 24 hours a day for the first few days. It can be removed to be washed or while you are taking a shower, eating, or cleaning the incisions. After the first week, you may feel more comfortable wearing this elastic band just at night for continued support during healing.

- You may shower and wash your hair gently with a mild shampoo 24–48 hours after surgery, or when you are comfortable doing so. Preferably, you should use a gentle, non-medicated shampoo such as Neutrogena or an antimicrobial wash such as Hibiclens during the first week after surgery.

- You should sleep with your head elevated on two or three pillows during the first two weeks following surgery. This helps with the swelling.

- You should keep a small amount of ointment along the incisions in front of the ear and the incisions in the crease behind the ear during the first week or two. In my practice, I recommend Aquaphor healing ointment. This will help keep the sutures moist and allow them to dissolve within approximately one week.

- If there is any crusting or dry blood on any of the face lift incisions, you may clean it with a Q-tip soaked in a mixture of equal amounts of hydrogen peroxide and water, or just plain water.

- You should avoid excessively turning your head or bending your neck for the first two weeks after surgery. When these maneuvers are necessary, you should move at the level of the waist by moving the shoulders and the head as one unit. This minimizes the pulling on the incisions and tissues.
- Eyeglasses may be worn as soon as the bandages are removed. However, you must ensure that the eyeglasses do not rest on or compress the incision lines around the ears.
- Most patients are able to use makeup after one week. You will need to avoid placing makeup directly over the incisions, but you should be able to place it over the rest of your face.
- You may resume brisk walking after two weeks, low-impact aerobics after four weeks, and complete normal activity after six weeks.

HOW LONG WILL THE FACE LIFT LAST?

- The face lift turns back the hand of the clock; it does not stop it. You begin to age again as soon as you leave the operating room table.
- On average, the changes accomplished with a face lift last 5–10 years. Depending on your skin characteristics, overall health, lifestyle, and whether or not you use maintenance regimens (Botox Cosmetic and soft tissue fillers), the effect of a face lift may be slightly longer or shorter.

ARE THERE ALTERNATIVES TO A FACE LIFT?

- There are adjuncts to "buy time." Although, these do not accomplish the tightening of the jowl and neck region achieved with a face lift, they may provide some changes that create a more youthful appearance. These include:
  - Soft tissue fillers to soften the nasolabial folds and fill out the cheeks or other areas of facial depressions
  - Botox injections to soften the wrinkles due to muscle contractions of normal facial expressions
  - Liposuction of the neck to address neck fullness
  - Laser treatment or chemical peels to address the fine, superficial wrinkles

WHEN IS THE RIGHT TIME FOR A FACE LIFT?

- Although everyone is different, as a general rule, the younger the patient, the less extensive the surgery. Older patients, or those with a heavy neck or thick skin, require more extensive surgery. Although there is no correct or incorrect answer to this question, it is reasonable to consider facial rejuvenation when there is evidence of skin laxity that begins to concern the patient. Usually, this occurs in patients in their 40s or 50s. At that time, the patient would benefit from a consultation to obtain information about appropriate future surgical and non-surgical facial rejuvenation procedures.

9

Neck Liposuction

WHAT IS NECK LIPOSUCTION, AND WHAT DOES IT ACCOMPLISH?

- Neck liposuction is the removal of fat from the neck region. Most of the fat in the neck is under the chin along the midline of the neck, and a lesser amount is found along the sides of the neck.
- In individuals with fullness along the neck due to fat deposits, liposuction gives the neck a more defined look. It improves the profile, often enhancing the chin and jaw definition.
- It is ideal in situations in which the neck skin has good elasticity and a slight-to-moderate amount of well-defined excess fat.
- Neck liposuction alone is not the procedure of choice when individuals have a significant amount of fat and excess skin along the neck. In these cases, liposuction of the neck often leads to redundancy of the skin, which creates its own concerns for the patient. In these situations, and in cases in which the patient starts out with redundant skin and fat along the neck, the skin needs to be lifted at the same time as the liposuction. This may be a limited lift or a more extensive one, depending on the amount and quality of the excess skin.

HOW IS NECK LIPOSUCTION PERFORMED?

- Three 3–4 mm incisions are made, one just behind the crease under the chin along the midline of the neck and one in the fold of skin attaching each earlobe to the cheek.

- Tumescent fluid (salt water containing medications to control bleeding and pain) is then infiltrated within the fatty layers of the neck.
- In some cases, a thin probe supplying ultrasound energy is introduced into the fatty layers to help break up the fat.
- Liposuction is then performed using a very small hollow metal tube (cannula) attached to a high vacuum.
- Using thinner cannulas helps to minimize the chance for irregularities along the surface of the skin.
- By using three incision sites, the liposuction cannula can be passed in a crisscross fashion along the entire neck region which further helps to minimize surface irregularities.
- Once liposuction is completed, the incisions are usually closed with dissolvable sutures and then covered with a piece of flesh-colored tape.
- After surgery, a compression dressing is placed to help the skin re-drape smoothly and to minimize swelling and bruising.

WHAT CAN I EXPECT AFTER NECK LIPOSUCTION?

- Most patients report very little pain after neck liposuction, but the area is tender to the touch. You will experience mild pressure from the dressings.
- The dressings are normally removed by the surgeon within the first few days after surgery and replaced with a face lift garment. This garment is worn for several days. You may remove it when showering or eating.
- During the first week after surgery, you will experience swelling and bruising of the neck. The compression garment helps to decrease the swelling.
- After approximately one week, the majority of the bruising and swelling will have subsided. But it will take on average approximately three to six months before you see the final results.
- The sutures are usually dissolvable and do not need to be removed.
- The scars, which measure approximately 3–4 mm in length, are well hidden and not easily seen.
- You should expect to have numbness along the neck, which begins to improve over the first few weeks after the procedure. It may not completely resolve for several months.

- You will have areas of firmness along the entire area that underwent the liposuction. This is due to the healing process occurring within the fatty layers under the skin. It resolves over a period of a few months.

HOW DO I CARE FOR MYSELF AFTER NECK LIPOSUCTION?

- As with all surgery of the head and neck, sleeping with your head elevated on two pillows during the first two weeks after surgery will help decrease the swelling and improve bruising following neck liposuction.
- The incision sites are usually covered with tape and do not require additional care.
- Pain medication is prescribed should it be necessary, but often patients do not require more than over-the-counter anti-inflammatory agents such as Tylenol.
- You may shower and wash your hair gently with a mild shampoo as soon as the initial surgical dressings are removed by the surgeon.
- You may begin to wear makeup as soon as you are comfortable doing so, but you should avoid placing makeup directly over the incisions until advised by your surgeon.
- As with a face lift, you should avoid excessively turning your head or bending your neck for the first two weeks after surgery. When these maneuvers are necessary, you should move at the level of the waist by moving the shoulders and the head as one unit.
- Most patients may resume completely normal activity after two weeks.

WHAT KIND OF ANESTHESIA IS RECOMMENDED FOR NECK LIPOSUCTION?

- Depending on the degree of liposuction necessary, the procedure may be performed under straight local anesthesia, or under local anesthesia with IV sedation (twilight anesthesia).
- In cases in which patients are very apprehensive, general anesthesia may be used.

10

Eyelid Lift (Blepharoplasty)

There are four main surgical procedures intended to rejuvenate the upper third of the face:

1. Upper blepharoplasty (upper eyelid lift)
2. Lower blepharoplasty (lower eyelid lift)
3. Transconjunctival lower blepharoplasty (Lower eyelid lift without a skin incision)
4. Brow lift

BLEPHAROPLASTY

The eyelids are structures that protect the eye from the external environment. They maintain moisture and lubrication of the eye and keep its surface free of debris to allow visual acuity. Over time, due to aging and genetic factors, the upper and lower eyelids develop changes in the skin, the underlying muscle, and the fat pads that surround the eye. These changes tend to make the individual appear tired or sad, and may give the area around the eye a puffy appearance (Fig. 10.1).

The changes occurring in the eyelids fall into four categories:

- Relaxation of the eyelid soft tissues, giving rise to the appearance of excess skin
- Protruding of the fat pads around the eye, giving rise to puffiness
- Hyperactivity of the muscles around the eye, giving rise to crow's feet
- Thinning of the eyelid skin, creating very fine, lacy wrinkles

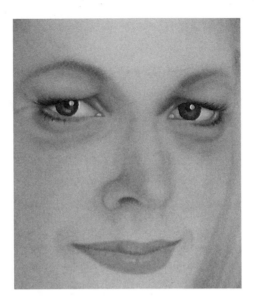

Figure 10.1.   As people age, the eyelid skin stretches, muscles weaken, and fat accumulates around the eyes, causing "bags" to form above and below the eye. (Courtesy American Society of Plastic Surgeons.)

Although all four of the above changes are occurring throughout the individual's lifetime, the order and rate at which they occur are usually related to genetic factors and lifestyle. Typically, when an individual presents for a cosmetic eye consultation, they have noticed the excess skin developing along the upper lid and the puffiness from protruding fat pads around the lower eyelid. However, the skin, muscle, and fat changes are occurring in both the upper and lower eyelids.

In general, there is usually more skin to remove from the upper eyelid than from the lower eyelid. Some patients develop puffiness of the lower lid without any changes in the skin itself. In these individuals, there is no need to remove skin from the lower eyelid, and they benefit from fat removal or fat repositioning alone. These are generally younger patients who are genetically predisposed to this fat pad herniation. They are candidates for a *transconjunctival blepharoplasty*, which will be discussed in detail later in this chapter. If the only concern is the presence of crow's feet, Botox Cosmetic may be used to soften the wrinkles without the need for surgery. If the concern is the fine, lacy pattern of wrinkles along the lower lids, surgery may not be benficial. These patients often think that they have "extra skin," but in reality they do not. The lacy wrinkles along the lower eyelids are due to the breakdown of collagen, and surgery will not add collagen. Usually, these patients benefit from skin-tightening procedures that stimulate the skin to make collagen, such as laser resurfacing or chemical peels.

What Is an Upper Blepharoplasty, and What Does It Accomplish?

- An upper blepharoplasty removes the excess skin and possibly fat from the upper eyelid. In addition to the removal of skin and fat, a strip of the muscle directly under the skin is removed to better sculpt the eyelid crease and to expose the two upper eyelid fat pads.
- An upper blepharoplasty provides more youthful eyelids and, if carefully performed, does not alter the shape of the eyes.
- In cases in which the lid appears heavy, an upper blepharoplasty allows the eyes to appear more open.
- In certain cases, the excess skin interferes with the individual's vision when looking upward. Surgery may improve this loss of visual field.

How Is an Upper Blepharoplasty Performed?

- The excess skin along the upper eyelid is marked. This is an elongated segment of skin extending across the entire eyelid from the inner corner of the eye to the outer corner of the eye. The lower limit of the marking is the natural eyelid crease. The upper limit of the marking is based on how much extra skin the patient has (Fig. 10.2). Care is taken to ensure that the patient can still close the eyes if the outlined segment of skin is removed.
- Once the outlined segment of the eyelid skin is removed, a thin strip (2–3 mm) of the underlying muscle is resected at the level of the eyelid crease along the full width of the eyelid.
- Pressure is then gently placed on the globe to evaluate the need to remove fat from the two fat compartments within the upper eyelid (Fig. 10.3). With pressure on the globe, any excess fat protrudes forward. If there is no protrusion of fat, then there is usually no need to remove any. If there is protrusion of fat, some is removed to prevent the upper eyelid puffiness. However, usually only a conservative amount of fat needs to be resected.
- The incision runs in the eyelid's natural crease and is closed with a nylon suture (Fig. 10.4).

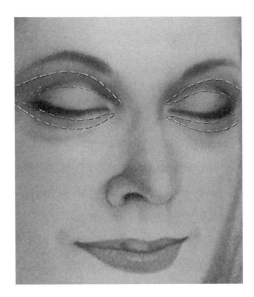

Figure 10.2. Before surgery, the surgeon marks the incision sites, following the natural lines and creases of the upper and lower eyelids. (Courtesy American Society of Plastic Surgeons.)

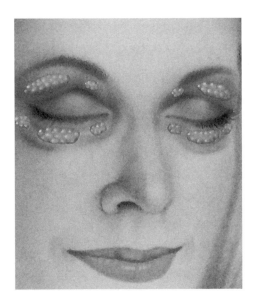

Figure 10.3. The underlying fat can be repositioned or removed during the surgery. (Courtesy American Society of Plastic Surgeons.)

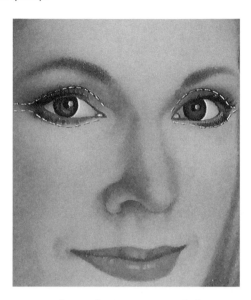

Figure 10.4. The surgeon closes the incisions with fine sutures, which usually leave very thin, nearly imperceptible scars. (Courtesy American Society of Plastic Surgeons.)

- Care must be taken to ensure that just the right amount of skin and fat are removed. Excess skin removal can result in the patient's inability to close the eye, resulting in chronic dry-eye symptoms. These can be significant and, at times, debilitating. Excess fat removal may make the eyelid appear hollow. This result often makes the individual have a sunken appearance to the eye.

Where Is the Incision for the Upper Blepharoplasty, and Are There Any Scars?

- The incision used to perform the surgery is placed within the skin crease of the upper lid.
- Although healing of any incision will result in a scar, the eyelid skin is very thin and consequently heals very well. In addition, the incision runs in the natural upper eyelid crease and, once healed, is usually not very visible.

What Is a Lower Blepharoplasty, and What Does It Accomplish?

- A lower blepharoplasty addresses the aging changes that occur within the lower eyelid.

- It improves the tired look by removing the "bags" and excess skin from under the eyes, giving a more rested and youthful appearance.
- The "bags" are due to protrusion of the lower eyelid's three fat pads. Although at times some of the fat needs to be removed, in many circumstances, it is repositioned. By repositioning and not removing the fat, the lower lid is not as likely to appear hollow with the passage of time.
- Usually, very little, if any, skin needs to be removed from the lower eyelid.

How Is a Lower Blepharoplasty Performed?

- Classically, a skin incision is placed directly under the lower eyelid lash line. This is carried through the underlying muscle to reach the lower eyelid fat pads (Fig. 10.2). The protruding fat is then evaluated (Fig. 10.3). It usually requires repositioning or, in some cases, a conservative resection. The extra skin is then removed, and the skin incision is closed with dissolvable sutures (Fig. 10.4).
- Many plastic surgeons prefer a technique that does not interrupt the muscle of the lower eyelid. In this method, the lower eyelid fat pockets are approached through an incision placed inside the lower eyelid, and any excess skin is removed through an incision placed directly under the lower eyelashes. The incision placed inside the lower eyelid does not need to be closed and heals well on its own. The skin incision may be closed with dissolvable sutures. Although this technique involves a little more work, it allows the muscle to remain undisturbed, thereby maintaining eyelid support and minimizing the potential for altering the eyelid position.
- The skin of the lower eyelid must be treated with great respect. There is very little room for error, and as such, skin excisions must be conservative. Excess skin excision from the lower eyelid results in a condition known as an ectropion, which is the pulling of the eyelid away from the globe. In minor cases, the lower eyelid is only slightly pulled down. In some cases, it can be detrimental with significant distortion of the eyelid position, necessitating surgical intervention to protect the eye itself and allow a more acceptable cosmetic appearance.
- Excessive excision of fat from the lower lid results in hollowness with a sunken appearance to the eyes. This may at times

create a worse and more aged appearance than the initial puffiness the patient wished to have addressed. In the past, lower eyelid surgery was approached by removing the protruding fat. Within the last decade, the trend has been to preserve as much of the fat as possible by repositioning it rather than removing it.

- More than any other structure in the face, the lower eyelid must be treated with caution and respect. It is very unforgiving to an aggressive approach.

Are There Scars with a Lower Blepharoplasty?

- Usually once the scars heal, they cannot be seen because the incision is placed behind the lash line.

LOWER TRANSCONJUNCTIVAL BLEPHAROPLASTY

What Is a Transconjunctival Blepharoplasty, and What Does It Accomplish?

- It is lower eyelid surgery that addresses the protruding fat through an incision made inside the lower eyelid (Fig. 10.5). All of the surgery is performed from inside the lower eyelid, without any external incisions.
- It treats the fat pads, or "bags," which cause one to look tired.

Who Is a Good Candidate for a Lower Transconjunctival Blepharoplasty?

- It is indicated for individuals who have puffiness along the lower eyelids without any associated excess skin. Since the puffiness is due to the bulging of the three fat pads, the excess fat may be repositioned or, in some cases, partially removed using an incision inside the lower eyelid without disturbing the overlying muscle or skin.

How Is a Transconjunctival Blepharoplasty Performed?

- Special shields are placed in the eye to protect the globe.
- An incision is made in the conjunctiva (the red portion inside the eyelid), and the three fat pads are gently teased and evaluated

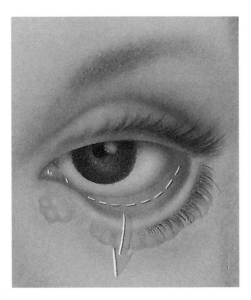

Figure 10.5. In a transconjunctival blepharoplasty, a small incision is made inside of the lower eyelid, and fat is repositioned or removed with fine forceps. No skin is removed, and the internal incision is closed with dissolving sutures or allowed to heal without sutures. (Courtesy American Society of Plastic Surgeons.)

(Fig. 10.5). They are then repositioned to provide a smoother contour along the lower eyelid. In cases in which there is a significant amount of fat, a small portion of the fat pads may need to be resected.

- In some cases, laser resurfacing of the skin may be combined with a transconjunctival blepharoplasty. This would tighten the skin and soften many of the fine wrinkles caused by breakdown of collagen. Laser resurfacing will be addressed in greater detail later in this section.

Are There Any Scars with a Transconjunctival Lower Blepharoplasty?

- No, the incisions are made inside of the eyelid. There are no incisions in the skin.
- If laser resurfacing is not performed, most people are presentable after three to five days. There may still be mild bruising that requires coverage makeup. If laser resurfacing is performed, recovery is at least 7–10 days.

Will I Be Awake during Eyelid Surgery?

- If an upper blepharoplasty is the only procedure being done, it may be performed under local anesthesia. If both an upper and lower blepharoplasty are being performed, twilight anesthesia is recommended. The majority of patients prefer this approach. If patients are extremely anxious, general anesthesia may be used.

What Can I Expect after a Blepharoplasty Surgery?

- Most patients will not experience significant pain from eyelid surgery. There may be some burning sensation for the first 24–36 hours that is usually relieved by cold compresses. You may take regular-strength or extra-strength Tylenol to alleviate this. Although pain medication is prescribed to ensure patient comfort, most patients report that there is very little pain.

- It is advisable to keep moist cool compresses on the eyes during the first 36 hours following surgery. This does not have to be continuous, but the longer that the cold compresses are in place, the more effective they will be. Rather than using ice packs, you may use gauze dipped in ice water and placed over the eyes. Once the gauze pads get warm, you should replace them. The moistened gauze is soothing to the incision and has the added advantage of absorbing any oozing (bleeding) from the incision line, thereby preventing crusting.

- There will be some initial bruising and swelling that develops over the first 24–48 hours. The cold compresses will help minimize this. In addition, you should keep your head elevated at least 30 degrees at all times during the day as well as at night when sleeping. This is easily accomplished by sleeping on two pillows. Doing so will help reduce the swelling that occurs.

- The bruising and swelling usually resolve over the course of two weeks, but there is a significant improvement of these symptoms within the first week. At times, bruising may work its way down into the cheek area. It is important to remember that there will be subtle swelling that is not obvious to others but noted by you and your surgeon for at least several weeks or, in some cases, months after surgery.

- Tearing and intermittent swelling are common for the first week and not uncommon for several weeks after surgery. Bruising around the eyes usually subsides within 7–14 days but can be covered with makeup by the end of the week. A small amount of blood may be seen along the eyeball itself, but usually this will clear without treatment. Occasionally, the lower eyelid will droop slightly during the first week or two as a result of swelling. If the eyes feel dry or irritated, you may use mild artificial tears. A list of the recommended eye drops is found at the end of this chapter.

• You may cover the upper eyelid incisions with a small amount of ointment at all times until the sutures are removed. With lower eyelid surgery, the incision under the eyelashes is usually closed with dissolvable sutures. These dissolve during the first week after surgery. To help these dissolve and keep the incision line free of any crusting, a small amount of ointment may be applied to the incision line. Many plastic surgeons prefer Ophthalmic Bacitracin ointment during this initial period after surgery. If you are allergic to Bacitracin, Tobradex Ophthalmic ointment is a good alternative.

• The prescribed ointment is used along the incision lines and if needed may also be placed as a lubricant inside the eye. Use of these ointments allows the incisions to remain adequately moisturized and optimizes the chance of a very fine scar. Often, patients return to their surgeon's office the day after their surgery to have the incisions cleaned. If you are not returning to the doctor's office the day after surgery, you may *gently* swab the incision lines with a Q-tip soaked in warm tap water. Your vision may become blurry due to ointment getting into the eyes, and it will take a couple of days for this to clear.

• With upper eyelid surgery, the sutures are not dissolvable and are usually taped to the nasal bridge and temporal regions with a small piece of skin tape. The sutures and skin tape should not be disrupted during the healing process, although ointment may be applied to the incisions.

• With lower eyelid surgery, there are approximately 6–10 small sutures underneath the lash line. Most surgeons use dissolvable sutures that dissolve over the course of the first week after surgery. To help keep the incisions moist and prevent crusting, you may apply a small amount of ointment to the incision line.

• You should avoid strenuous activities during the first two weeks following surgery to minimize the chance of bleeding and subsequent bruising. These include such activities as bending, stooping, heavy lifting, or strenuous sports. For exercise, you are encouraged to walk at a leisurely pace.

- Two weeks after surgery, you can begin increasing your activity level as tolerated. It is advisable to wait approximately four weeks before resuming heavy aerobics, jogging, weightlifting, or extreme exercises, which cause a great deal of straining.

- Small whiteheads may occur along the incision line in either the upper or lower eyelids. These are not unusual and can be easily removed in your doctor's office.

- You may wear makeup everywhere except along the eye area immediately after surgery. In most circumstances, it is possible to wear eye makeup after one or two weeks.

- Although you may feel well enough to return to work within a day or two after surgery, you will still be bruised and swollen at that time. For purposes of privacy, most patients return to work after one week. Even then, some may still require coverage makeup for any residual bruising.

LASER RESURFACING

Many lasers are used today for a variety of conditions, such as sun damage, scars, skin discoloration, and undesirable hair as well as wrinkles. Lasers may be simply classified into *ablative* and *non-ablative* types. The ablative lasers remove the outside layer of the skin, leaving a raw surface that requires healing. The non-ablative lasers do not affect the outer layer of the skin, but work at a deeper level. There is usually very little or no downtime following treatment with the non-ablative lasers. A thorough discussion of all types of lasers requires its own textbook. Consequently, we will only address the Erbium YAG laser. This is an ablative laser used to treat wrinkles and has become the gold standard (replacing the carbon dioxide laser) against which all other ablative and non-ablative skin rejuvenation lasers are compared.

How Does the Erbium YAG Laser Resurfacing Improve Wrinkles?

- The energy from the laser removes the outer layers of the skin and stimulates collagen formation. Since many of the fine lines and wrinkles are due to collagen breakdown in the skin, formation of new collagen diminishes the appearance of these fine lines.

- Although Erbium YAG laser resurfacing may be used throughout the face for the treatment of fine lines, it is especially useful around the eyes. The thinner skin of the eyelids responds well to the collagen stimulation effect of the laser energy.

- Laser resurfacing may be performed by itself or along with eyelid surgery.

- If laser resurfacing is to be used around the eyes, the use of Botox Cosmetic in that area two weeks prior to the laser procedure minimizes the movement of the muscles that give rise to the crow's feet. This has the advantage of minimizing the movement of the skin around the eyes during the healing period, thereby giving the new skin a smoother surface on which to build. Although this practice is used by many, the use of Botox Cosmetic around the eyes is considered an off-label use (see Chapter 15).

What Are the Major Risks of Laser Resurfacing?

- The primary risks with laser resurfacing are the potential for scarring and the potential for loss of pigment (hypopigmentation) or darkening (hyperpigmentation) of the lasered area.

Who Are Good Candidates for Laser Resurfacing?

- In general, individuals with fair and thin skin are the best candidates in terms of both improvement of wrinkles and lower risk of pigment changes. The darker the skin, the greater the potential for pigment changes. The thicker the skin, the less improvement in the extent of wrinkles.

How Do I Take Care of Myself after Laser Resurfacing?

- There are many ways of managing lasered patients after their procedure. Surgeons vary greatly in the approach that they use. Some believe in keeping a dressing over the area to prevent contact with the environment, and some believe in keeping the area uncovered so it may be cleaned and observed continuously. I have managed all of my laser patients with the latter technique. It has resulted in rapid healing without scarring or infection and has resulted in minimal pigment changes. However, it is important to note that the technique described here is only one approach, and you must follow the directions given by your physician.

Open Technique

- It is important to keep the lasered areas clean and moist.
- The lasered areas will feel like a sunburn. Cool, moist compresses may help with that sensation.
- In the first 24 hours, you need to keep a thick coat of Aquaphor ointment over the entire area. This ointment protects the raw surface of the skin and prevents drying. Cold compresses may be applied above the layer of Aquaphor.
- If there are areas of bleeding, you may gently clean these using cotton balls or Q-tips soaked in cold saline. Then, immediately reapply the Aquaphor ointment.
- In the first 48 hours, use cool saline gauze over the lasered area. Water will sting the raw skin. Some patients feel greater comfort by spraying cool saline over the lasered area. After the first 48 hours, you may use cool water. Be certain to reapply the Aquaphor ointment immediately after the cool compresses are removed in order to prevent dryness of the lasered skin.
- Two days following the laser procedure, you may begin washing your face gently with tap water or saline. Do not use any soap or facial cleansers at this time. Use your fingertips or cotton balls to wash, and be very gentle. Following the cleansing, apply a thick coat of Aquaphor ointment over the lasered area.
- You need to keep a thick layer of Aquaphor ointment over the lasered area at all times. Expect to repeat the application of the ointment every couple of hours while awake, and whenever you wake up in the middle of the night, until the lasered area stops oozing.
- During the first week, continue to gently cleanse the area 5–6 times a day, and continue to reapply Aquaphor ointment. It is important to keep the resurfacing areas covered with a thick coat of ointment at *all* times to avoid crusting or drying.
- *Never pick at crusts that do not loosen easily.* This could lead to scarring. Apply the ointment and cool compresses to them, and they should come off easily with time.

What Can I Expect after Laser Resurfacing?

Each case is different, and some people may heal faster than others. The following are general guidelines for the Erbium YAG resurfacing laser:

- The intense pink color will fade within 5–7 days, and a light pink will replace it for several days up to several weeks.

- Patients who are prone to have cold sores (fever blisters) may have a flare-up following resurfacing. Most plastic surgeons place patients on anti-herpetic medications such as Zovirax or Valtrex as a precaution to help prevent this. It should be noted that the prophylactic use of anti-herpetic medications in this fashion is considered an off-label use. If you should happen to develop blisters, notify your surgeon immediately so that he or she may prescribe the necessary treatment.

- Occasionally, small "whiteheads" may appear in the treated areas; these usually disappear within two to three weeks, but occasionally take longer. They should not be manipulated, except by your physician.

- After the first week of healing, the skin will still feel somewhat tense and dry. I generally recommend using the prescribed Aquaphor ointment at night and Eucerin cream or lotion during the day. Do not use anything else without first checking with your physician.

- In most cases, makeup may be used to cover the pink color of the treated areas after 10–14 days.

- Generally, you may be able to return to school or work as soon as the weeping has subsided. Around the eyes, the weeping usually stops within five to seven days. It may take two to three days longer if other areas of the face were treated. Although the weeping will have subsided at this time, you will still have an intense red or pink color.

- The skin will retain swelling for several weeks following laser resurfacing. It is important to be patient, since continued improvement in the texture of the skin may occur up to 6–12 months in some cases.

- You should avoid direct sun rays for at least three months, since your "new" skin will be more sensitive and will have a tendency to burn and tan more easily. You should protect the resurfaced areas with a sunscreen product for three to six months, and you should wear a large brimmed hat to shade the face during this interval. The sun screen preparation should have an SPF of 45 or greater.

- You should avoid prolonged exposure to the sun (sunbathing, golfing, fishing, tennis, or similar activities) during the sunny parts of the day throughout the first three to six months.
- If the resurfaced area should start to turn brown, you need to notify your physician immediately, as you may need to be treated with an anti-pigmentation cream.
- If you should develop increased redness, or increased pain or ulcerations, around the lasered area, you need to notify your physician immediately, as these may be signs of a serious infection.

ARTIFICIAL TEARS RECOMMENDED FOLLOWING EYELID SURGERY

- Bion Tears Lubricant Eye Drops
- Celluvisc Lubricant Eye Drops
- GenTeal Eye Drops
- HypoTears PF Lubricant Eye Drops
- Moisture Eyes
- Ocucoat PF Eye Drops
- Refresh Tears
- Tears Naturale Forte
- TheraTears Lubricant Eye Drops

11

Brow Lift

WHAT IS A BROW LIFT, AND WHAT DOES IT ACCOMPLISH?

- It is a surgery that lifts the brow, the temples, and the middle of the forehead.
- If the eyebrows have drooped and the upper eyelids look heavy, a brow lift can elevate the brows and give the eyes a more youthful, open look.
- It will make the eye area look more alert and less heavy.
- It can also *partially* correct brow asymmetry if one eyebrow is drooping or sagging more than the other. No one is symmetrical, and perfect facial symmetry is not a realistic goal.
- It can remove folds of skin by the bridge of the nose if they are caused by drooping of the forehead skin. This is especially true in individuals with very thick skin.
- A brow lift also addresses the forehead wrinkles. These include the horizontal wrinkles across the upper forehead and the vertical wrinkles in between the eyebrows (Fig. 11.1).
- Often, a brow lift is used in conjunction with an upper blepharoplasty to help rejuvenate the brow and upper eyelid region. Each of these two procedures accomplishes a different goal. An upper blepharoplasty reduces the excess skin and puffiness of the upper eyelid without changing the position of the eyebrow or affecting the appearance of the forehead. A brow lift lifts the eyebrows, creating more distance between the lash line and the eyebrow. It relaxes many of the forehead wrinkles and gives the appearance of less skin along the upper eyelid.

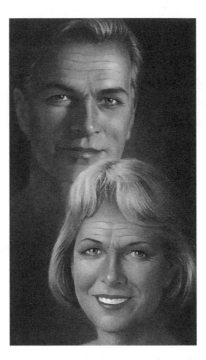

Figure 11.1. A brow lift addresses the horizontal wrinkles across the forehead and the vertical wrinkles in between the eyebrows. (Courtesy American Society of Plastic Surgeons.)

- Two approaches may be used to achieve a full brow lift. The approach used depends upon the patient's individual needs and the surgeon's expertise. These two approaches include:
  - Coronal brow lift
  - Endoscopic brow lift

How Is a Coronal Brow Lift Performed?

- This is the older of the two procedures and still has appropriate indications and uses.
- An incision is made along the hair-bearing scalp from the upper aspect of one ear across the scalp to the upper aspect of the other ear (Fig. 11.2).
- The soft tissues of the entire forehead are then elevated from the underlying bony attachments.

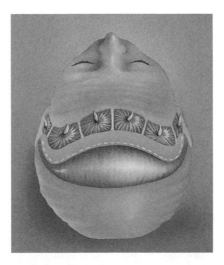

Figure 11.2. The incision for a coronal brow lift extends across the scalp, usually behind the hairline. (Courtesy American Society of Plastic Surgeons.)

- This dissection continues all the way from the scalp incision to the level of the eyebrows.
- Once the eyebrows are released from the underlying bone, the first portion of the procedure is complete.
- The second part of the procedure approaches the forehead muscles. Some of the muscle fibers are cut or gently teased out to weaken the muscles, thereby softening the forehead wrinkles.
- Finally, the soft tissues of the entire brow are then lifted upward, elevating the brow and eyebrows to the desired position.
- The excess skin that results from the elevation process is then removed (Fig. 11.3).
- This procedure may shift the hairline back a bit. In individuals with a low hairline, this may be desirable. In individuals with a high hairline, the central aspect of the incision may have to be placed just at the junction of the hairline and forehead skin to prevent shifting the hairline back.
- The coronal brow lift is the preferred approach in individuals who have either redundant forehead skin that needs to be removed, or significantly thickened forehead muscles that require a more aggressive resection than is possible with an endoscopic brow lift. In most other cases, surgeons favor the endoscopic brow lift.

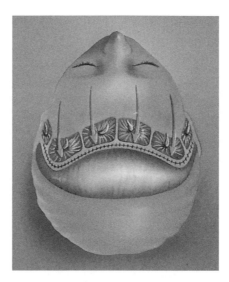

Figure 11.3.   After the forehead muscles that create the wrinkles are weakened or partially removed, the brow is lifted to a more desirable position, the excess scalp tissue is removed, and the scalp incision is closed with sutures. (Courtesy American Society of Plastic Surgeons.)

How Is an Endoscopic Brow Lift Performed?

- An endoscopic brow lift does not require the extensive incision used in the coronal brow lift.
- It uses special thin, long instruments and a very small, thin camera to accomplish similar goals.
- In this technique, three or four ½-inch incisions are made in the scalp just behind the hairline. These are positioned in such a way as to allow the surgeon access to work under the skin and muscles of the forehead.
- The camera is placed through one of these incisions, and the endoscopic surgical instruments are placed through the other incisions to elevate the forehead soft tissues from the underlying bone and to release the necessary muscles. The camera guides the surgeon so that he or she can see the muscles, vessels, and nerves during the surgery, and can safely accomplish the necessary dissection under direct visualization.
- Once the skin and muscles are released form the underlying bony attachments, some of the muscle fibers are cut or teased out to soften the forehead wrinkles.

- The soft tissues are then lifted upward and tightened to elevate the brows and forehead.
- Usually, skin is not excised with an endoscopic brow lift, and there is a much lower chance of shifting the hairline.

DOES A BROW LIFT HURT?

- Most patients report a pressure-type pain with an associated headache during the first two days following surgery.
- The majority of patients indicate that the pain is significantly relieved after the first 24–48 hours.

ARE THERE SCARS WITH A BROW LIFT?

- The endoscopic brow-lift incisions are placed in the hair-bearing scalp and heal well. They are usually covered by the patient's hair and are not easily visible.
- If the coronal brow lift incision is placed behind the hairline, it also heals well and is covered by the patient's hair.
- If the central part of the coronal incision is placed at the junction of the hairline and scalp to prevent shifting of the hairline, the incisions along the upper forehead are initially quite visible. Typically, these heal very well and are far less noticeable after they have lost their red color. However, they are permanent. This is an important note for individuals who wear their hair pulled back, as they may need to modify their hairstyle after surgery.

WHAT TYPE OF ANESTHESIA IS RECOMMENDED FOR A BROW LIFT?

- Since most of the dissection is performed deep to the level of the muscle, general anesthesia is recommended for both types of brow lift procedures.

WHAT CAN I EXPECT AFTER A BROW LIFT?

- When you wake up in the recovery room, you will have a dressing over the surgical site. Most surgeons wrap a head dressing across the forehead and scalp immediately following the brow-lift surgery. This is worn during the first few days after surgery in order to minimize swelling and bruising.

- Expect the first night to be uncomfortable, with a feeling of tightness and pressure along the forehead and scalp. This is usually due to both the surgery and the dressing. Pressure-like or throbbing headaches are common. The prescribed pain medication will help control the discomfort.

- It is not uncommon for some patients to experience nausea during the first 24 hours following surgery. It is a good idea to discuss the potential for nausea with your surgeon prior to surgery so that the appropriate medications may be prescribed for use after your procedure.

- After the first night or two, the majority of discomfort will have subsided, and most patients will require only non-narcotic pain medication such as Tylenol.

- Expect to have some bruising and swelling around the eye region. It takes approximately one week for the majority of the swelling and bruising to resolve. You may have residual bruising and swelling for up to two or three weeks after surgery.

- You may experience a band-like tightness across the forehead. Much of this improves within the first two to four weeks after surgery. However, it is not uncommon to experience subtle tightness during the first three months after surgery.

- Immediately after surgery, you will have swelling and numbness in front of the ears as well as across the forehead. Usually the majority of the swelling subsides in one to two weeks, and the numbness improves over the course of three to six months.

- Once the initial swelling has resolved, you may still have some residual fullness or a feeling of hardness along the forehead and in front of the ears. This is a natural consequence of the healing process, and these areas will soften over a period of three to six months.

- You may have subtle irregularities along the skin surface of the brow immediately after surgery. These are usually secondary to swelling and resolve over the first few weeks as the swelling decreases.

- On average, it takes approximately one week to feel comfortable performing most normal activities.

- Most surgeons use dissolvable sutures. These fall out within 7–10 days. Under some circumstances, removable sutures will be used, and these are usually removed within 7–10 days after surgery.

HOW DO I CARE FOR MYSELF AFTER A BROW LIFT?

- In the first 24–48 hours, you may place an ice pack over the forehead dressing and cold compresses over the eyes. These may be alternated on and off as comfort permits, usually every 15 minutes. Using cool packs and compresses will help diminish the swelling and bruising.

- As with any facial surgery, you should sleep with your head elevated on two pillows (approximately 30 degrees) during the first two weeks after surgery. This helps minimize the swelling and allows it to resolve faster.

- You may shower and wash your hair gently with a mild shampoo when the dressing is removed. It is best to avoid medicated or heavily fragrant shampoos. You may use Johnson's Baby Shampoo or Hibiclens Skin Cleanser during the first week after surgery.

- You should avoid hair spray, mousse, gels, and styling products during the first two weeks after surgery, since they may be irritating to the fresh incisions.

- You need to be very cautious using hair dryers and curling irons during the first two weeks after surgery. Since you will not have normal sensation along the scalp, it will be difficult to appreciate the extent of heat generated with these items, and consequently, you may accidentally burn your scalp.

- You should avoid hair coloring for approximately four weeks after surgery, depending on how you are healing.

- Most physicians use absorbable sutures. You may find it comfortable to cover the incisions with a small amount of Aquaphor ointment. This will keep the sutures moist and allow them to dissolve within the first 7–10 days following surgery. If there is any crusting or dry blood on any of the incisions, you may clean it gently in the shower or with a Q-tip soaked in water.

- You may wear eyeglasses as soon as the bandages are removed. However, you must be careful to ensure that the eyeglasses do not rest on the incision lines around the ears.

- You may wear makeup immediately over the face as long as the incisions are avoided.

- You may increase your activity level as tolerated. You may resume brisk walking after two weeks, low-impact aerobics after four weeks, and complete normal activity after six weeks.

HOW LONG WILL A BROW LIFT LAST?

- As with a face lift, lifestyle and genetics influence the rate at which we age, and consequently affect the longevity of these cosmetic procedures. Usually, a brow lift will last 5–10 years.

12

Nose Surgery (Rhinoplasty)

WHAT IS A RHINOPLASTY, AND WHAT DOES IT ACCOMPLISH?

- A rhinoplasty is the surgical correction of the nose. The word "rhino" comes from the Greek word "rhinos," which means "nose," and the word "plasty" comes from the Greek word "plastikos," which means "to mold."
- A rhinoplasty addresses any or all of the structures within the nose, including the bones, cartilage, skin, and fatty tissues.
- The nose holds a very significant position in the face. Not only is it in the center, but it also projects from the face. Consequently, a large or prominent nose can overcome the face and easily draw attention away from the other features.
- Being a linear, unpaired structure in the middle of the face, the nose is expected to follow a straight line. Any deviation from that expected symmetry is more easily detectable by the human eye than it is with the other facial features.
- A rhinoplasty may be performed exclusively for cosmetic purposes, functional purposes, or both (Fig. 12.1). It may achieve any or all of the following:
  - Restore the airway to allow improved breathing
  - Reduce asymmetries and improve alignment
  - Decrease excess height, width and length of the nose
  - Provide better definition along the nasal tip
  - Lift a drooping nasal tip

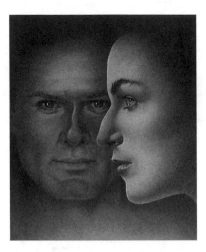

Figure 12.1. Before surgery, these rhinoplasty patients have large, slightly hanging noses, with a hump and an enlarged tip. (Courtesy American Society of Plastic Surgeons.)

- Decrease flaring of the nostrils
- Create a nose that is more proportional and in better harmony with the other facial features

HOW IS A RHINOPLASTY PERFORMED?

- In general, rhinoplasty procedures may be classified into one of two types: open rhinoplasty or closed rhinoplasty.
- The primary difference between the two is that the open rhinoplasty requires a very small incision along the vertical segment of tissue separating the two nostrils (columella).
- Usually, the more extensive or complex rhinoplasty procedures are approached through an open technique.
- In both approaches, the skin and soft tissues are elevated from the underlying cartilage and bone. These structures are then trimmed or, in some cases, augmented to the appropriate dimensions (Figs. 12.2a, b). The nasal bones may be broken to achieve improved alignment (Figs. 12.3a, b). Once the changes have been made to the cartilage and bone, the skin and soft tissues are allowed to re-drape over the new framework (Fig. 12.4).
- Thinner skin is more likely to re-drape over the new framework and allow the changes within the bone and cartilage to manifest.

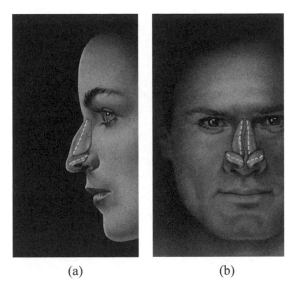

Figure 12.2a, b. Incisions are made inside the nostrils or at the base of the nose, providing access to the cartilage and bone, which can then be sculpted into shape. (Courtesy American Society of Plastic Surgeons.)

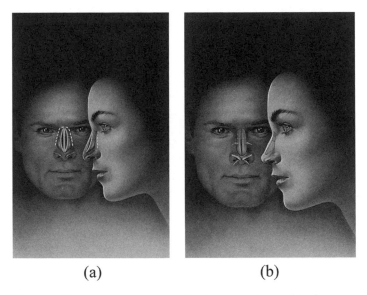

Figure 12.3a, b. The surgeon removes the hump using a chisel or a rasp, then brings the nasal bones together to form a narrower bridge. Cartilage is trimmed to reshape the tip of the nose. (Courtesy American Society of Plastic Surgeons.)

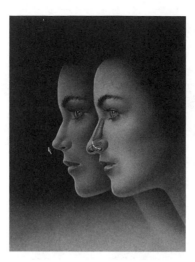

Figure 12.4.   Once the bone and cartilage have been modified, the skin is allowed to re-drape over the new framework. (Courtesy American Society of Plastic Surgeons.)

In general, thinner skin is more favorable in rhinoplasty procedures than thick skin. However, excessively thin skin is unforgiving, and any slight irregularities in the cartilage or bone may be visible externally.

- Thick skin does not re-drape back as easily as thin skin. This can pose limitations in the changes that may be achievable with a rhinoplasty. This is especially true along the nasal tip, where thick skin can significantly limit the extent of achieving tip refinement and definition.

WHERE ARE THE INCISIONS PLACED?

- In a closed rhinoplasty, all incisions are placed inside the nostrils.
- In an open rhinoplasty, the majority of the incisions are placed inside the nostrils, but a small incision is placed along the vertical strip of skin separating the nostrils (columella) to allow better visualization of the underlying structures. This external incision generally heals very well and is usually not easily perceptible once completely healed.
- If the patient needs narrowing or reshaping of the nostrils, an incision is placed at the base of each nostril to excise some of the

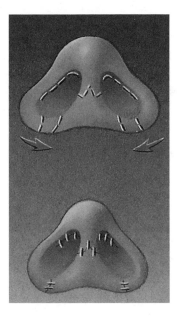

Figure 12.5. If your nostrils are too wide, the surgeon can remove small wedges of skin from their base, thereby creating smaller nostrils. (Courtesy American Society of Plastic Surgeons.)

skin and soft tissues (Fig. 12.5). The incision is hidden within the crease at the junction of the nostril and the cheek, and it is not usually visible once healed. This approach may be used with both the closed and open rhinoplasty procedures.

WHAT IS THE RECOVERY TIME?

- Most patients feel well after the first two to three days following surgery.
- If the bones were broken to realign them, a small cast (nasal splint) is kept along the upper three-fourths of the nose to stabilize the bones. This usually stays in place for one week.
- If the nasal bones are not broken, rhinoplasty patients can return to work as early as three to five days following their procedure because they feel well. However, they will still have significant swelling and some bruising at that time.
- If the nasal bones are broken, patients experience more discomfort, swelling, and bruising and will be wearing the nasal splint

during the first week following surgery. In these cases, most patients do not return to work until after one week.

- The majority of the bruising resolves after two weeks.
- The majority of the swelling subsides in the first six weeks; however, there is a slight degree of swelling, especially along the nasal tip, that can persist up to one year.

WHAT KIND OF ANESTHESIA IS RECOMMENDED DURING A RHINOPLASTY?

- Depending on the degree of surgical correction necessary, the procedure may be performed under local anesthesia with IV sedation (twilight anesthesia), or under general anesthesia.
- In extensive rhinoplasty cases, or when patients are very apprehensive, general anesthesia is recommended.

DOES A RHINOPLASTY HURT?

- All patients experience an aching sensation along the nose during the first two to three days following a rhinoplasty.
- If the nasal bones require breakage, there will be more pain than when the surgery is limited to the nasal cartilage and soft tissues.
- Normally, all pain is reasonably controlled with the prescribed pain medication.

ARE THERE ANY SCARS?

- In a closed rhinoplasty, all of the scars are inside the nose. They are not noticeable to the patient unless they become thick and create a problem with breathing.
- In an open rhinoplasty, the only external scar is along the vertical strip of skin separating the nostrils. This is placed carefully and is not usually easily perceptible. As with the closed rhinoplasty, the remaining scars are all inside the nose.
- In individuals who require reduction or reshaping of the nostrils, there may be a scar within the crease between each nostril and the cheek. Since these scars are within the crease, they are usually very well hidden and not easily seen.

WHAT CAN I EXPECT AFTER RHINOPLASTY?

- When you awaken in the recovery room, you will have some discomfort along the entire nasal area. If the bones were broken, you will have more pain than if the procedure involved the cartilage and soft tissues only. The nasal splint (small cast) will be in place across the upper three-fourths of the nose (Fig. 12.6). There will be a small gauze pad taped beneath the nostrils (moustache dressing) to catch any bleeding that might occur. It is normal for this gauze pad to accumulate blood and require multiple changes during the first 24 hours following surgery.

- You may experience a headache, especially if the septum was treated or the nasal bones were broken. A mild or moderate headache is not unusual. However, if the headache is severe or the worst headache that you have ever experienced or if it does not resolve after the first 24–48 hours, you need to notify your surgeon. If some of the nasal bones are addressed to improve the airway (the bones that form part of the septum or the turbinates which are the bones along the internal sidewall of the nose that help regulate airflow), a severe headache may signify injury to the bone plate that separates the nose from the brain. This is a very rare complication, but one that is worthy of mention.

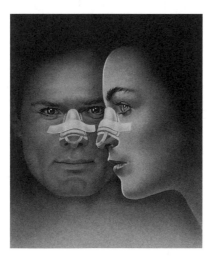

Figure 12.6. A splint made of plastic, metal, or plaster is applied to the nose during the first week after rhinoplasty to support the bone and cartilage in their new shape during the initial healing period. (Courtesy American Society of Plastic Surgeons.)

- You will have swelling and bruising. Both will become worse over the first 48 hours after surgery.
- The swelling occurs along the nasal tip, both eyes, and the forehead. The only part of the nose that is not noticeably swollen is the part covered by the nasal splint, as this provides pressure and minimizes swelling.
- The bruising will accumulate around your eyes.
- Expect to have an aching sensation in the nose for the first few days following surgery. The prescribed pain medication is sufficient to alleviate the pain.
- You should not experience any excessive bleeding. If you have bleeding that cannot be contained within the small gauze pad under the nose, you should call your surgeon immediately.
- If the nasal bones were broken, there is the potential to develop numbness along the sides of the nose and part of the cheek, due to sacrificing certain branches of the nerves close to the line of fracture. This numbness may be temporary or permanent.
- Due to swelling, you may be unable to breathe through the nose for several days. If this is uncomfortable, you can begin using a nasal spray such as Afrin or Neo-Synephrine, or a nasal decongestant such as Sudafed tablets, during the first week after surgery. The spray should only be used for three to four days, since longer usage may lead to a rebound effect, making the nose more congested.
- The nasal splint and tape will be removed approximately one week following surgery. When the splint is removed, you will see the new shape of the nose. There will be a fair amount of swelling through the nasal tip as well as across the bridge. This subsides in the first two to three months following surgery. It will take approximately *one year* to see the final appearance of the nose. The changes that occur over this long period of time are subtle and will be noticed by you and your surgeon. However, the average acquaintance or family member may not notice the change in swelling as it occurs.
- In cases of open rhinoplasty, the small incision along the skin separating the nostrils (columella) will be slightly pink at the time the splint and tape are removed. During the first four to six weeks after surgery, it is helpful to keep this incision covered with an ointment such as Aquaphor. This serves to provide a moist environment for the new scar and allows the potential for faster healing.

- Once the swelling has decreased, you may be able to feel some irregularities along the nasal bridge. This is a natural consequence due to the healing of the underlying bone and cartilage. These irregularities are usually felt, but on rare occasions, may also be seen. In more extreme cases, patients may develop a small bump along the bridge of the nose. This is usually the result of a callous along the nasal bones that forms during the healing process. In some cases, this requires a secondary surgery to address it.

HOW DO I CARE FOR MYSELF AFTER RHINOPLASTY?

- Sleeping with your head elevated by using two pillows as well as staying upright during the day will help reduce the swelling more quickly.
- You may place cold compresses (ice pack) over the eyes and across the bridge of the nose during the first 36–48 hours following surgery. The compresses should be left on for 15 minutes and taken off for 15 minutes, or as comfort permits.
- You will have a small gauze pad taped beneath the nostrils (moustache dressing) to catch any bleeding that might occur. You will need to change this gauze pad several times during the first 24 hours following surgery.
- The nasal splint will remain in place for approximately one week. The nasal splint is resistant to water, but can come off if it accidentally gets wet or becomes dislodged. You need to be careful not to disturb the placement of the splint, since it may affect the stability of the nasal bones.
- You may shower and wash your hair the day following surgery. You should keep your back to the shower to avoid getting the splint wet. Once out of the shower, you should gently pad the face dry while avoiding the nasal splint.
- Once the splint is removed, you should avoid wearing sunglasses or reading glasses, since these will cause an imprint along the bridge of the nose. If the eyeglasses are absolutely necessary and seem to be creating an imprint, you may choose lighter glasses or tape the glasses to the forehead to prevent any compression of the nose. You may wear contact lenses as soon as it is comfortable for you to do so.
- You should avoid contact sports for the first three months following surgery to avoid reinjuring the nose. After three months, the

nasal bones will have healed and would need to be re-broken for damage to be done.

- If you are exposed to the sun, it is advisable to wear sunscreen with an SPF of 45 or greater during the first three to six months following surgery to avoid a sunburn to the nose. This is especially important in cases in which there are external incisions along the nose, such as in open rhinoplasty or when the base of the nose has been resected to reduce the size of the nostrils. If the external incisions are exposed to the sun before they are completely healed, they may become darker (hyperpigment).

- Most plastic surgeons prescribe antibiotics, especially when extensive work has been done to the nose. It is very important that you take the prescribed antibiotic to help prevent infection.

- Most plastic surgeons will see their patients the day after surgery to evaluate their progress and remove any potential packing. The nostrils are gently cleaned at that time.

- If you are not returning to see your surgeon the day following surgery, you may clean your nose at home. This is done by gently swabbing the crusted areas with a Q-tip saturated with warm water. Once all of the scabs have been gently loosened and removed, you may cover the internal and external incisions with an ointment, such as Aquaphor. This will help minimize crusting along the incisions and will aid in the healing process.

- With rare exceptions, all sutures are dissolvable and do not require removal. As the sutures dissolve, they will fall out of the nostrils and the external skin incisions. The sutures are clear, thin pieces of thread resembling light, fine hairs.

- All external incisions will be slightly pink during the first several weeks. You may wear makeup over these two weeks after surgery or when the incisions are no longer crusting.

HOW LONG WILL THE EFFECT OF THE RHINOPLASTY LAST?

- Although a rhinoplasty accomplishes permanent changes in the nose, it is normal to expect the nose to change with age, even in individuals who have never had nasal surgery.

- As we age, we lose fat throughout our face, including the nose. Similarly, the natural loss of bone and decrease in the strength of supporting structures leads to drooping of the nasal tip.

- The extent to which these changes become noticeable depends upon the starting point of the nose in terms of bony support, thickness of the skin, and prominence of the cartilage. The thinner the skin and the more prominent the cartilage, the more noticeable these changes will become.

WHEN IS THE RIGHT TIME FOR A RHINOPLASTY?

- A rhinoplasty may be performed in an adult of any age. Those over 50 or 60 years of age may have slightly more brittle bones and thinner skin than younger patients, but they can usually undergo a rhinoplasty quite successfully.
- In very young patients, it is safe to consider a rhinoplasty once the face has completed growing. Usually, facial features reach their adult proportions after completion of puberty. As such, it is safe to consider rhinoplasty in girls after 14 or 15 years of age and in boys after 15 or 16 years of age.

13

Facial Implants: Chin, Mandibular, and Cheek Implants

WHAT ARE CHIN, MANDIBULAR, AND CHEEK IMPLANTS?

- Most facial implants are made out of a soft, solid form of silicone. Other types include a solid, porous (spongelike) material, which allows the surrounding scar tissues to grow into the implant, thereby limiting its potential movement.
- Chin implants are placed along the front surface of the jawbone to increase projection in individuals with a receding chin (Fig. 13.1).
- Mandibular implants are placed along the side surface of the jawbone to provide a wider and more defined jawline (Fig. 13.1).
- Cheek implants are placed along the cheekbones to provide better projection and contour of the cheeks in individuals lacking definition in the midface (Fig. 13.1).
- With all three types of implants (chin, mandibular, and cheek), the facial bones and teeth must be studied very carefully prior to surgery. The first step is evaluating the relationship of the upper teeth to the lower teeth and how they fit together. This relationship is referred to as "occlusion." Occlusion of the teeth is a very important consideration in evaluating a person's facial profile. If the teeth do not fit together, the individual needs a more extensive workup to determine the cause of this poor alignment. After evaluation of occlusion, the relationship of the upper facial bones to the lower facial bones needs to be examined. Often, a chin that is perceived as being deficient may be due to a more major deficiency of the entire jaw. This is not a condition that is simply addressed with a chin or mandibular implant and often requires more extensive

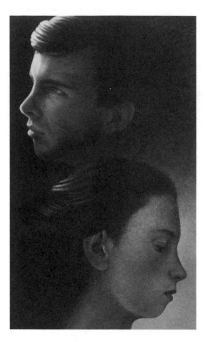

Figure 13.1.   Facial implants may be used in individuals with a receding chin, decreased projection of the cheeks, or a poorly defined jawline. (Courtesy American Society of Plastic Surgeons.)

jaw surgery. Also, a chin may be small due to lacking projection and vertical length. In these situations, an implant may not provide a cosmetically acceptable appearance. Similarly, a perceived lack of projection along the cheekbones may actually be due to an overly projecting jaw or chin. In these situations, the jaw alone or the jaw and cheek bones need to be addressed.

WHAT DOES A CHIN IMPLANT ACCOMPLISH?

- It provides increased projection of the chin in order to improve the individual's profile.
- It is a very good procedure for those who simply have a recessed chin.
- In general, a chin implant provides increased chin projection, but it cannot provide increased length to the chin in cases in which there is a vertical deficiency. A sliding genioplasty (to be discussed later in this chapter) is considered in these cases.

- There are several shapes and styles of chin implants depending upon the individual's needs.
- With the use of a chin implant, patients can enhance the profile of the chin, widen the chin, or produce a different contour altogether.

HOW IS CHIN IMPLANT SURGERY PERFORMED?

- Most surgeons insert the implant through a small incision (approximately three-fourths of an inch) placed directly behind the crease under the chin. This incision is well hidden and usually heals very nicely. Although some surgeons will use an incision inside the mouth, the incidence of infection is slightly higher in these circumstances, and as such, the external incision is usually favored.
- Once the incision is made, the soft tissues along the front surface of the jawbone are elevated (lifted off the bone) to create a pocket that approximates the shape and size of the desired implant.
- The chin implant is then inserted into this pocket directly on top of the underlying jawbone (Fig. 13.2).

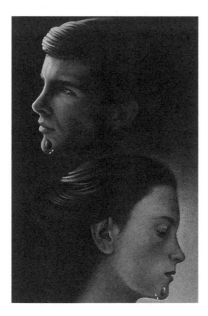

Figure 13.2. Chin implant position and incision for placement. (Courtesy American Society of Plastic Surgeons.)

- The implant may be anchored with stitches to the adjacent soft tissues in order to minimize chances of it shifting during the initial healing period.
- The incision is then closed in multiple layers to provide adequate soft tissue coverage over the implant. The skin incision is usually closed with dissolvable sutures and covered with surgical tape to protect it during the healing phase.
- Some surgeons favor additional immobilization of the implant during the first week of healing by the use of external taping to hold it in place.

WHAT DOES A MANDIBULAR IMPLANT ACCOMPLISH?

- Mandibular implants provide increased width to the jaw, thereby creating a stronger and smoother jawline.
- This is a good procedure for those who have normal facial proportions but simply need better definition along the jaw.
- There are several shapes and styles of mandibular implants, depending upon the individual's needs.
- Caution must be used with mandibular implants. Often, a narrow jaw is associated with a deficiency in the overall size of the jaw. These cases must be addressed by a thorough evaluation of how the upper and lower teeth fit together, and the size discrepancy of the jaw relative to the rest of the face. In some cases, the deficiency requires expansion or surgical widening of the jawbone.

HOW IS A MANDIBULAR IMPLANT SURGERY PERFORMED?

- Most surgeons insert mandibular implants through two small incisions (approximately one inch each in length) placed inside the mouth. Each incision is made within the recess between the lower gums and cheek tissue on the two sides of the jaw.
- Once the incisions are made, the soft tissues overlying the jawbone are elevated (lifted off the bone) to create a pocket that approximates the shape and size of the selected mandibular implant.
- The implants are then inserted into their respective pockets directly on top of the underlying jawbone (Fig. 13.3).

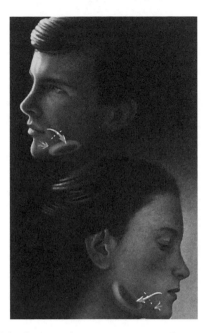

Figure 13.3. Mandibular implant position and incision for placement. (Courtesy American Society of Plastic Surgeons.)

- As with chin implants, mandibular implants may be anchored with stitches to the adjacent soft tissues in order to minimize chances of it shifting during the initial healing period.
- Each incision is then closed in multiple layers to provide adequate coverage over the implant.

WHAT DO CHEEK IMPLANTS ACCOMPLISH?

- Cheek implants provide projection along the cheekbone and/or the area just below the cheekbone known as the "submalar region."
- They are a nice alternative for individuals who lack projection or who do not have good definition of the cheek area.
- Cheek implants help to define and shape the upper third of the cheek region. In doing so, they also lift the soft tissues along the lower cheek, providing a more youthful look to the middle one-third of the face.

HOW IS CHEEK IMPLANT SURGERY PERFORMED?

- The first step in planning cheek implant surgery is to determine the most appropriate position for the implant along the cheek region. Should the placement be directly over one area of the cheekbone, or should it be along the cheekbone and the region below it?
- Once the best position is determined, the shape and size of the implant is selected.
- Most surgeons insert cheek implants through two small incisions (each approximately one inch in length) placed inside the mouth. Each incision is made within the recess between the upper gums and cheek tissue on the two sides of the face.
- Once the incisions are made, the soft tissues overlying the cheekbones are elevated (lifted off the bone) to create a pocket that approximates the shape and size of the selected implant.
- Each implant is then inserted into its respective pocket directly on top of the underlying facial bones (Fig. 13.4).

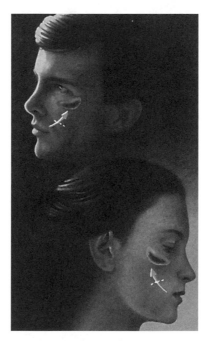

Figure 13.4. Cheek implant position and incision for placement. (Courtesy American Society of Plastic Surgeons.)

- As with the other two types of facial implants discussed, cheek implants may be anchored with stitches to the adjacent soft tissues in order to minimize chances of shifting during the healing period. Shifting of cheek implants can lead to significant asymmetry.
- Each incision is then closed in multiple layers to provide adequate soft tissue coverage over the implants. Usually, dissolvable stitches are used.
- As with chin and mandibular implants, some surgeons favor additional immobilization of the cheek implants during the first week of healing by the use of external taping.

WHAT IS THE RECOVERY TIME FOLLOWING CHIN, MANDIBULAR, OR CHEEK IMPLANT PROCEDURES?

- Most patients require three to five days following implant placement to feel comfortable.
- There is a mild bruising and moderate swelling that persists for the first two to four weeks following surgery. At that time, most patients continue to have a very mild swelling that is perceptible to the patient and their physician, but not to the general public. It can take 6–12 months for the final swelling to subside.

DOES FACIAL IMPLANT SURGERY HURT?

- In cases of a chin or mandibular implants, the chin, the lower gums, and jawline are sore for approximately one week.
- In cases of cheek implants, the upper gums, cheeks, and temple areas are painful during the first week.
- The majority of the pain subsides after the first three days, and becomes mild for the rest of the week.
- Eating a soft diet and speaking as little as possible helps to decrease the discomfort.
- Pain medication is always prescribed and should be taken for comfort.

WHEN ARE THE SUTURES REMOVED?

- Usually, dissolvable sutures are used for all incisions inside the mouth. If non-dissolvable sutures are used for external chin implant incisions, they are typically removed at five to seven days after surgery.

ARE THERE ANY SCARS WITH CHIN IMPLANT PLACEMENT?

- If the chin implant is placed using an external approach, there is an approximately ¾-inch scar under the chin that is placed behind the natural crease and, consequently, not easily visible.
- If the chin implant is placed through an incision inside the mouth, there is no external scar.

ARE THERE ANY SCARS WITH CHEEK OR MANDIBULAR IMPLANT SURGERY?

- No. Since cheek and mandibular implants are usually placed through incisions inside the mouth, there are no external scars.

WILL I BE AWAKE DURING SURGERY?

- Chin, mandibular, and cheek implants may be placed under IV sedation (twilight anesthesia), with the patient partially asleep. Otherwise, the procedure may be performed under general anesthesia so that the patient is completely asleep.

WHAT CAN I EXPECT AFTER FACIAL IMPLANT SURGERY?

- When you initially awaken from chin or mandibular implant surgery, expect to have a sensation of mild pressure and pain along the chin, lower gums, and jawline. When you awaken from cheek implant surgery, the sensation of pressure and pain is along the cheeks, temples, and upper gums. This aching sensation diminishes over the first few days following implant surgery and is controlled with the prescribed pain medication.
- You may have tape across the jaw for a chin or mandibular implant, and across the cheeks for a cheek implant, during the first five to seven days after surgery. This tape helps to further immobilize the implants and protect them from shifting. It must remain in place until removed by your surgeon at your postoperative visit.

- When the tape is removed, you will see the new shape of your chin, jawline, or cheeks. There will be a fair amount of swelling throughout the jawline in the case of chin or mandibular implants, and the cheekbones in the case of cheek implants.

- For approximately one week, you will have extensive swelling and moderate bruising.

- After the first week following chin or mandibular implants, you may think that the chin looks "boxy" or "square" due to the swelling. Similar swelling is seen after cheek implants, giving rise to wider features along the cheeks and midface. The swelling will gradually fade over a period of two to four weeks.

- Although most of the swelling resolves during the first three months after surgery, it may take another six to nine months or longer for the remainder of the swelling to resolve. The changes that occur over this long period of time are subtle. They will be far less noticeable to other people than they will be to you and to your surgeon.

- Once the swelling has decreased, you may be able to feel the edges of the implant(s). This is a natural consequence of the healing process and requires no treatment.

HOW DO I CARE FOR MYSELF AFTER FACIAL IMPLANT SURGERY?

- You should keep an ice pack on the area of the implant for the first 36 hours following surgery. It is comfortable to alternate the ice pack on and off every 15 minutes.

- It is very important to take the prescribed antibiotic to help prevent infection.

- It is best to sleep on your back with your head elevated on two pillows for the first two weeks. Staying upright during the day will also help reduce the swelling more quickly.

- It is uncommon to experience significant bleeding after facial implant surgery. If you experience any bleeding that does not subside with mild pressure, you must notify your surgeon immediately.

- You may bathe and wash your hair the day after your implant surgery. If there is tape over the chin, jaw, or cheek area, it must not get wet.

- A soft diet is recommended during the first one to two weeks after surgery.

- You should refrain from facial movements that may shift the implants, such as excessive smiling or kissing, during the first two weeks after surgery.
- You should not manipulate the implants during the first three months after surgery to minimize the potential for shifting. In fact, during this early period, you should avoid contact sports or activities that could potentially traumatize the surgical area and alter the position of the implant(s).
- If you notice any significant asymmetry in your jawline or cheeks, you should notify your surgeon immediately.
- If you notice a recurrence of the pain along the teeth after the pain had resolved, it may indicate that there is pressure from the implant along the roots of the teeth due to shifting of the implant. In these cases, you need to notify your surgeon.
- If the chin implant was placed using an external incision, the incision beneath the chin will be slightly pink at the time the tape is removed. This will fade over the course of 6–12 months. As with any external scar, you need to avoid sun exposure and wear sunscreen with an SPF of 45 or greater until the scar has completely faded. Otherwise, it may develop a dark color that does not fade well over time. The incision may also feel more comfortable if covered with an ointment such as Aquaphor during the first two to four weeks after surgery.
- If the chin implant was placed using an incision inside the mouth, and in cases of mandibular and cheek implants, which are usually placed through an incision inside the mouth, you need to keep the incision clean at all times. This necessitates washing the mouth with a medicated mouthwash after all meals and snacks. You may also feel more comfortable if you adhere to a soft diet during the first week after surgery until the incisions have completed the initial stages of healing.
- You may wear makeup as soon as you are comfortable doing so. You need to be cautious when applying makeup in the region of the implants during the first two weeks after surgery, so as to avoid excessive pressure and potential shifting.

HOW LONG WILL THE FACIAL IMPLANTS LAST?

- Although chin, mandibular, and cheek implants are placed with the expectation that they will last a lifetime, they may not.
- The implants may shift, become infected, or become exposed.

- If an implant shifts, it can create an asymmetry or impinge on facial nerves or the roots of the teeth.
- If the implant shifts, it must be adjusted surgically.
- If the implant becomes infected or exposed, it must be removed. It may be replaced after complete resolution of the infection. Most surgeons wait several weeks prior to replacing the implant under these circumstances.

ARE THERE ALTERNATIVES TO CHIN IMPLANT SURGERY?

- For individuals who wish to avoid a chin implant, a sliding genioplasty is a possibility.
- A sliding genioplasty involves cutting the central and lower part of the jawbone and sliding it forward and, if needed, downward. The incision is along the inside of the mouth, in the recess between the gums and lower lip.
- For individuals who have a small chin that is deficient in projection and length, a chin implant is not an ideal solution, as it will only provide increased projection.
- In cases in which there is a need to increase both projection and length, a sliding genioplasty is generally a more appropriate solution than a chin implant.
- In less common conditions in which the chin projects too much, a sliding genioplasty may be performed to set the chin back to create a softer profile.
- The recovery time following a sliding genioplasty is longer than that with a chin implant, but the goals are different. A sliding genioplasty avoids the potential for future changes associated with an implant, such as shifting, exposure, or infection. From a cosmetic standpoint, a sliding genioplasty allows advancement of the muscles attached to the anterior aspect of the chin. Not only can this impact the facial profile, but it can also improve the neck contour.

WHEN IS THE RIGHT TIME TO CONSIDER A FACIAL IMPLANT?

- When patients present for chin, mandibular, or cheek implants, it is important to be certain that their facial growth is complete and that the upper and lower teeth and jawline are in normal positions relative to one another and relative to other facial bones.

- If the perceived small chin is due to abnormalities in the relation-ship of the upper teeth to the lower teeth, or in the relationship between the teeth to other facial bones, this condition must be addressed prior to considering any type of chin implant or genio-plasty. Similarly, if the perceived lack of facial projection along the cheeks is associated with excessive or deficient projection of the jaw, placement of cheek implants may not be appropriate.
- In these situations, it is best for patients to be evaluated by maxillofacial and plastic surgeons, who can assess the face using special studies called *cephalometric analyses*. These studies measure the relationship of the lower jaw and upper jaw to each other and to the rest of the face, and they help guide the best course of action.

14

Ear Surgery (Otoplasty)

WHAT IS AN OTOPLASTY?

- An otoplasty is a surgical procedure to reshape the ear.
- Different techniques and approaches are available to address congenital abnormalities of the ears or to restore damaged ears.
- It is beyond the scope of this book to address all of the potential conditions of the ear requiring surgical correction and their respective procedures. Most of the time, individuals seek an otoplasty to set back prominent ears that project too much from the side of the head (Fig. 14.1). This is the condition that will be addressed in this chapter.

WHAT DOES AN OTOPLASTY ACCOMPLISH?

- When the ears are prominent, usually two structural components are contributing to this prominence.
  - The ear lacks the appropriate folds along its surface.
  - The ear projects too much from the side of the head.
- An otoplasty reshapes the ear cartilage and repositions it to create more natural folds within the ear. It also corrects the position of the ear relative to the side of the head.

HOW IS AN OTOPLASTY PERFORMED?

- First, the patient is examined to determine if one ear (unilateral), or both ears (bilateral) are affected.

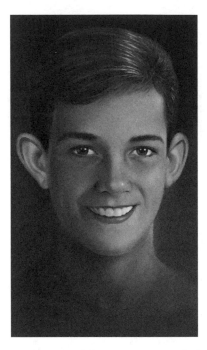

Figure 14.1. Ears that appear to stick out or are overly large can be helped by an otoplasty. (Courtesy American Society of Plastic Surgeons.)

- The affected ear is analyzed to determine what aspects are deficient or missing, and what aspects are excessive.
- Once the treatment is determined, a longitudinal elliptical or dumbbell-shaped incision is made along the back of the ear, in the small recess of skin between the ear and the side of the head.
- The skin and soft tissues are then elevated from the underlying cartilage, and the cartilage is folded to create the typical folds found within the normal human ear. Special stitches are used to hold the new folds in place (Fig. 14.2). If the cartilage is thick and solidified, it may not bend easily. In these situations, the cartilage may be gently thinned with a special device (dermabrasion machine) to permit improved molding.
- After the necessary folds are created in the cartilage, the ear is then pinned back to the side of the head using additional stitches to hold the ear cartilage in place (Fig. 14.3).
- After the ear is pinned back, the skin behind the ear is evaluated, and the redundant skin and soft tissue is removed.

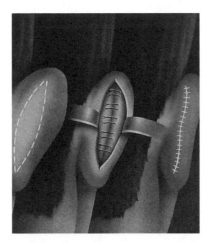

Figure 14.2. An incision is made in the back of the ear so cartilage can be sculpted and folded as needed. Stitches are used to help maintain the new cartilage shape. (Courtesy American Society of Plastic Surgeons.)

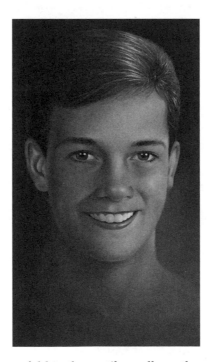

Figure 14.3. Creating a fold in the cartilage allows the ear to lie closer to the head and be much less prominent. (Courtesy American Society of Plastic Surgeons.)

- Only under rare circumstances is there a need to cut away or remove cartilage. What appears to be overgrown cartilage in a prominent ear is corrected once the appropriate anatomical folds of the ear cartilage are created.
- If cartilage is cut, it usually creates sharp edges that distort the smooth transitions seen in the folds of the natural ear.
- The skin incision is then closed with dissolvable stitches.
- The ears are dressed with a fitted dressing to protect their new shape and position. The goal is to prevent forward displacement of the ears while they heal. Most surgeons prefer to have this dressing stay in place for four to five days after surgery. Following this early period, patients may still need to protect the repair by wearing a removable headband over the ears.

WHERE ARE THE INCISIONS PLACED?

- With very rare exceptions, all incisions may be placed in the crease behind the ear, and consequently will not be easily visible.

WHAT IS THE RECOVERY TIME FOLLOWING AN OTOPLASTY?

- The initial recovery takes approximately one week. Patients may resume work and activities of daily living after the initial four to five days. However, the final shape of the ear may not be completely apparent for 6–12 months following surgery.

DOES AN OTOPLASTY HURT?

- There is a mild pain for the first few days after surgery, often described as a throbbing throughout the ear. There is also a pressure-like pain behind the ears. Some patients report a generalized headache.
- The outer aspect of the ears is often numb during the initial healing period. This may take weeks to months to resolve.

WHEN ARE THE SUTURES REMOVED?

- Usually, dissolvable stitches are used to close the skin incision behind the ear.

- If non-dissolvable stitches are used, the ear would have to be displaced forward to remove the stitches. This maneuver may disrupt the newly pinned back position of the ear.

WHAT KIND OF ANESTHESIA IS RECOMMENDED DURING AN OTOPLASTY?

- Depending on the patient's age and comfort level, twilight anesthesia (local anesthesia with sedation) or general anesthesia may be used.
- Young children and anxious adults would be best served with general anesthesia, whereas others have an option between the two types.

WHAT CAN I EXPECT AFTER AN OTOPLASTY?

- When you wake up in the recovery room, you will have a band-like head dressing wrapped around the ears. This dressing usually has a special mold to protect the new shape of the ear cartilage, and it provides slight pressure to decrease the swelling in the ears during the initial healing process. It is important that this dressing remains undisturbed; if it slips, it must be reapplied by the surgeon.
- There is minimal bleeding associated with this procedure. It would be unusual to see any blood soaking through the dressing. If a small amount of blood stains the dressing, you should not be alarmed. However, if the blood stain continues to increase in size, you need to contact your surgeon.
- The pain is generally mild and relatively equal on both sides. If you experience excessive pain on one side relative to the other, it may be an indication of bleeding. This requires evaluation by your surgeon immediately.
- If there is minor bleeding under the skin following an otoplasty, your surgeon may be able to remove it by simply using a needle and syringe. In cases in which it is more extreme, it will require evacuation in the operating room.
- Your dressing will usually be removed four to five days after surgery. Once the dressing is removed, expect your ears to be swollen and bruised. Although the appearance of the ears at this point will give some indication as to the final result, they will look far more natural over the subsequent two weeks.

- You may experience some numbness along the outer edge of the ears for the first two to three months. This is normal and results from cutting across some of the small nerves that provide sensation to the skin. Over time, these nerves regrow, and sensation should be fully recovered. It may take up to one year for complete return of sensation. There is rarely permanent numbness.

HOW DO I CARE FOR MYSELF AFTER THE OTOPLASTY?

- You may clean the crease behind the ear by using a Q-tip soaked with tap water. The sutures placed behind the ears will dissolve within one to two weeks and do not need to be removed.
- During the first four weeks, you should apply a small amount of ointment, such as Aquaphor, to the incisions once or twice daily. This will help to protect the incisions as they heal.
- Usually, there is only mild pain following an otoplasty. If you experience significant pain that is not relieved with the prescribed pain medication, you need to notify your surgeon.
- It is very important to take the prescribed antibiotic to help prevent infection.
- During the first two weeks following surgery, you should sleep on your back with your head elevated on two pillows to help decrease swelling. You should also avoid strenuous activity. This includes bending, stooping, heavy lifting, aerobic exercises, or strenuous sports.
- During the first six to eight weeks following surgery, you should avoid contact sports, since an inadvertent blow to the ear may disrupt the repair. You may resume full activity after this period of time.
- After removal of the dressing, you will need to wear a headband over the ears when sleeping. The purpose of this band is to hold the ears back in their new position. In doing so, the band reduces some of the initial tendency that the cartilage may have to slip back into its old position. It also prevents the ears from being accidentally pulled forward during sleep. Many surgeons recommend wearing the band while sleeping for a period of three to four months following surgery. It may be worn longer if you feel comfortable doing so.
- Rarely, a stitch in the cartilage will become irritated or become exposed through the incision behind the ear. This may happen

within the first month, or it may happen as late as several years following your surgery. If a stitch does extrude through the skin, it is a simple procedure to address in your surgeon's office.

HOW LONG WILL AN OTOPLASTY LAST?

- In general, an otoplasty achieves the cartilage shape changes required for long-term benefit. However, cartilage has memory, and there is potential that the repair may not hold, allowing the prominent ear to recur. In fact, recurrence of prominent ears is not uncommon.

WHEN IS THE RIGHT TIME FOR AN OTOPLASTY?

- The ideal time to perform an otoplasty for correction of prominent ears is during childhood, as the ears are nearly fully developed by five to six years of age.
- From a social and psychological standpoint, most surgeons recommend performing an otoplasty prior to the child attending school in order to avoid possible potential social ridicule by other children.
- Many people do not seek repair of prominent ears until adulthood. Generally, no additional major risks are associated with ear surgery in adults; however, the cartilage is usually thicker and firmer in these patients. The surgical outcome of an otoplasty in both children and adults is very successful.

Non-Surgical Approaches
to Facial Rejuvenation
and Enhancement

15

Botox Cosmetic

WHAT IS BOTOX COSMETIC?

- Botox Cosmetic is a highly purified muscle-relaxing agent that is derived from the bacterium Clostridium Botulinum.

- It is also known as Botulinum Toxin Type A and belongs to a group of drugs known as neurotoxins.

- There are seven different types of Botulinum toxins (Type A, B, C, D, E, F, G). Each has its own unique properties and effects. Botulinum Toxin Type A is Botox Cosmetic, and it is the most widely studied of all types.

- Botulinum Toxin Type A has been safely used in the fields of neurology and ophthalmology for many years. It is approved by the Food and Drug Administration (FDA) for the treatment of eyelid spasm and muscle spasm causing crossed eyes, as well as for correcting one-sided facial muscle spasm.

- Botox Cosmetic gained general acceptance in the field of cosmetic surgery in 2003, when it received approval by the FDA for cosmetic treatment of the wrinkles in between the eyes. Although this has remained as the only FDA-approved cosmetic indication, most physicians use Botox Cosmetic to treat wrinkles in many other parts of the face. These uses are considered off-label uses.

- Botox Cosmetic injections are the most common cosmetic procedure performed today.

HOW DOES BOTOX COSMETIC WORK?

- Botox Cosmetic causes a temporary relaxation of the muscle into which it is injected.
- Botox Cosmetic acts at the level of the nerve-muscle junction to prevent muscle contraction.
- Normally, the motor nerves in the body stimulate the movement and contraction of specific adjacent muscles. The nerve sends a message to the muscle to induce its contraction. This message is "transmitted" to the muscle by a "neurotransmitter" known as acetylcholine. When acetylcholine is released from the nerve into the adjacent muscle, the muscle receives the message to contract.
- Botox Cosmetic enters the nerve ending and blocks the release of this neurotransmitter, acetylcholine. Consequently, the muscle does not get the message to contract and is temporarily paralyzed.

WHAT DOES BOTOX COSMETIC ACCOMPLISH?

- Years of muscle contraction have an effect on the skin that is attached to these muscles. As the muscles contract repeatedly over many years, the attached skin is being pulled repeatedly according to the direction of the muscle contraction. Since each muscle will contract in only one direction, the pull on the skin is only in one direction. This leads to creases and wrinkles in the skin that follow a predictable pattern. Initially, these wrinkles and creases are present only when you are making a particular expression and contracting a particular muscle. Eventually, with years of repetitive movement, the wrinkles become etched into the skin and are visible even when your face is at rest. For example, the smile lines around the eyes become noticeable when we smile in our 20s or 30s. With repetitive smiling, these wrinkles eventually become etched in the skin, leading to persistent crow's feet.
- Botox Cosmetic softens or prevents wrinkles and creases by limiting the ability of the underlying muscles to contract.
- The only FDA-approved use of Botox Cosmetic is in the treatment of the vertical lines in between the eyebrows. All other uses that will be discussed are considered off-label uses.

- Botox Cosmetic is most commonly used to treat the vertical creases in between the eyebrows caused by frowning, the creases across the forehead due to raising the brows, and the crow's feet that develop from smiling (Figs. 15.1, 15.2). The use of Botox Cosmetic has also extended to the lower third of the face and the neck. Although this is not as common as use in the upper third of the face, Botox Cosmetic is being used to treat wrinkles around the lips, decrease deep nasolabial folds, soften prominent neck bands, and lift the downward turn of the corner of the mouth that occurs with aging.

- Generally, Botox Cosmetic is very useful in the upper one-third of the face, and the combination of Botox Cosmetic with soft tissue fillers is useful in the lower third of the face. Soft tissue fillers will be discussed in Chapter 14.

- Botox Cosmetic gives the face a smoother and softer appearance by improving existing wrinkles and slowing down the formation of new wrinkles.

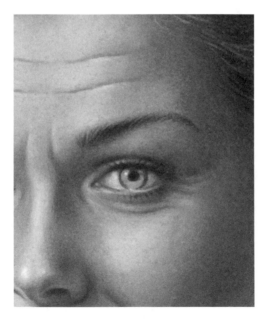

Figure 15.1. Over time, the natural facial expressions that we make result in wrinkles in the upper third of the face. These are due to muscle movement and occur in a predictable pattern. (Courtesy American Society of Plastic Surgeons.)

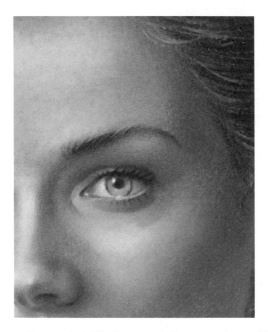

Figure 15.2.   Botox Cosmetic is FDA-approved to treat frown lines in between the eyes. Off-label uses include the forehead wrinkles and crow's feet. (Courtesy American Society of Plastic Surgeons.)

HOW IS IT DONE?

- A small needle is used to inject a very small amount of Botox Cosmetic into the muscles that are causing the wrinkles. Several injections are given per specific muscle.
- There is a slight stinging sensation that lasts a few seconds after the injection. Ice is helpful with the discomfort.
- Botox Cosmetic may begin working as early as 24 hours after injection and may take up to two weeks to reach its full effect.

HOW LONG DOES THE EFFECT OF BOTOX COSMETIC LAST?

- Injection of Botox Cosmetic into the small muscles causes those specific muscles to halt their contraction temporarily. Each individual's response to Botox Cosmetic depends upon their own metabolism of the drug.

- In general, the therapeutic effect of Botox Cosmetic will last approximately three months. Consequently, most people require Botox Cosmetic injections four times per year in order to maintain its effect.

WHAT CAN I EXPECT IMMEDIATELY AFTER THE BOTOX COSMETIC INJECTIONS?

- Generally, there is minimal recovery following Botox Cosmetic injections.
- The injection session lasts only a few minutes.
- You will have slight stinging at the injection site, but this lasts only a few seconds.
- You may experience very mild redness and swelling at the injection site for several minutes after the injection.
- If you have a tendency to bruise, ice is helpful.
- You may apply makeup almost immediately after the injections.
- Patients undergoing any kind of injection procedures should try to abstain from products that increase bleeding. A listing of these products is found in the Appendix.
- If there is slight bleeding at the site of the injection, you may gently apply pressure to it.

WHAT ARE THE SIDE EFFECTS AND POTENTIAL RISKS FOLLOWING BOTOX COSMETIC INJECTIONS?

- Although Botox Cosmetic is safe to use repeatedly, every product has potential side effects. In general, Botox Cosmetic treatments have very limited risks or complications.
- There have not been any reported cases of systemic toxicity from accidental injection or oral ingestion of Botox Cosmetic.
- The effect of Botox Cosmetic may be altered by certain antibiotics (aminoglycosides) or other drugs that interfere with neuromuscular transmission. Consequently, a thorough review of the patient's medical history, including their daily medications, is crucial.
- Complications are rare, but may include paralysis of nearby muscles, headaches, flu-like symptoms, local numbness, rash, bruising, and activation of herpes zoster (in patients who carry this virus).

- Although any muscle adjacent to the injection site may be temporarily paralyzed by Botox Cosmetic, the results are temporary and will resolve.
- If injected to treat the wrinkles in between the eyes or along the forehead, Botox Cosmetic may cause a temporary drooping of the eyelid or drooping of the forehead, respectively. There are prescription eye drops (Iopidine) available to correct the eyelid drooping until the full Botox Cosmetic effect has dissipated.
- If injected for treatment of prominent nasolabial folds (off-label use), Botox Cosmetic may cause a temporary vertical lengthening of the upper lip by relaxing the adjacent muscles that normally elevate the lip border. If this occurs, a soft tissue filler substance may be injected into the lip to help elevate the border.

CAN REPEAT INJECTIONS OF BOTOX COSMETIC DIMINISH ITS EFFECT OVER TIME?

- Infrequently, repeat injections of Botox Cosmetic may be associated with decreased efficacy. Usually, the longer one uses Botox Cosmetic, the longer the benefits. So, why does it have a diminished effect in some people over time?
  - Botox Cosmetic contains very small amounts of proteins. When these proteins enter the human body, the natural response is to form antibodies to them. After they are formed, these antibodies attack the Botox Cosmetic proteins when they enter the body, making Botox Cosmetic less effective.
  - The likelihood of forming antibodies is reduced by having treatments no more frequently than is necessary to achieve the desired result. Treatments with Botox Cosmetic should not be administered until the effect of the previous treatment has diminished. In general, this is approximately every three months.
  - The cumulative dose of Botox Cosmetic should not exceed 200 units in a 30-day period. Fortunately, this is a high number of units and is not normally exceeded with cosmetic applications of Botox Cosmetic.

WHO IS NOT A CANDIDATE FOR BOTOX COSMETIC INJECTIONS?

- Active inflammatory skin reactions such as herpetic blisters, rashes, or hives necessitate postponing Botox Cosmetic injections until the condition has resolved.

- Women who are pregnant, attempting to become pregnant, or breast feeding should avoid Botox Cosmetic, since its safety during these conditions has not been established.
- The safety of Botox Cosmetic injections has not been established in individuals 12 years of age or younger.
- Patients with certain neuromuscular diseases (diseases that involve nerves and muscles) should avoid Botox Cosmetic. These include:
  - Amyotrophic lateral sclerosis (ALS)
  - Motor neuropathy
  - Neuromuscular junctional disorders
  - Myasthenia gravis
  - Lambert-Eaton syndrome
- Patients with neuromuscular disorders may be at increased risk of the systemic effects of Botox, including difficulty swallowing and breathing.
- Serious and/or immediate hypersensitivity (allergic) reactions have rarely been reported. These reactions include:
  - Itching
  - Hives
  - Soft tissue swelling
  - Difficulty breathing
- Options for alternative treatment may include injection of fillers or the surgical excision of the muscles, depending on the area in question.

16

Soft Tissue Fillers

As we age, the changes that occur in our face are a manifestation of the effects of gravity, sun damage, hereditary influences, and loss of volume. The change in volume is due to loss and redistribution of fat within the face, thinning of the skin dermis (deep layer of the skin), and bone loss. All of these changes lead to: descent of the forehead, the eyebrows, and the cheeks; downward turning of the corners of the mouth; thinning of the lips; drooping of the nasal tip; prominence of the folds along the sides of the nose and mouth (nasolabial folds); greater visibility of the bony structures; and an overall relaxation of the soft tissues seen as jowls and redundant tissue along the neck.

Injectable soft tissue fillers consist of a group of natural or synthetic substances that restore volume within the facial skin and the deeper tissues, giving rise to a fuller, more youthful appearance. As of 2010, there are many injectable soft tissue fillers that have been FDA-approved for cosmetic use in the United States. These include Zyderm, Zyplast, Cosmoderm, Cosmoplast, Restylane, Perlane, Hylaform, Hylaform Plus, Captique, Prevelle Silk, Juvederm Ultra, Juvederm Ultra Plus, Radiesse, and Sculptra Aesthetic. Zyderm and Zyplast are forms of bovine collagen, while Cosmoderm and Cosmoplast are forms of human collagen. Restylane, Perlane, Juvederm Ultra, Juvederm Ultra Plus, Hylaform, Hylaform Plus, Captique, and Prevelle Silk are all forms of hyaluronic acid. Radiesse is a calcium-based product, and Sculptra Aesthetic is a synthetic filler consisting mostly of Poly-L-Lactic acid.

Each of these soft tissue fillers will be addressed individually and in detail later in this chapter. There are other fillers available that are not FDA-approved. These will not be addressed. Caution must be exercised when considering treatment with any product or procedure that is not FDA-approved. The FDA has strict guidelines to ensure the

proper use of various therapeutic modalities. Improper or unap-
proved use may lead to significant complications. Patients must be
very judicious in the treatment modalities they seek and the physicians they seek to perform them.

All currently available and FDA-approved soft tissue fillers are
temporary in nature. They must be repeatedly injected into the tissues
to maintain their effect. The length of time they remain in the soft tissues varies with the characteristics of the filler itself, the area of the
face into which the filler is injected, and the patient's unique response
to the filler.

Most patients who seek treatment with soft tissue fillers often wonder why there is not an FDA- approved injectable permanent filler.
Although the concept of "permanent correction" of soft tissues may
seem very attractive, it is important to remember that our specific
facial features are not "permanent." With aging and weight fluctuations, our facial features undergo significant change. As such, a soft
tissue filler that may have appeared perfectly placed at one point in
life may be very misplaced in the future, as the facial features shift
due to the natural forces of aging or weight change. Furthermore, permanent fillers may have long-term side effects, such as migration,
asymmetry, and lumpiness. In these situations, permanent fillers are
very difficult to remove, since they are not an implant, but an injection.
Consequently, it is much safer to use temporary soft tissue fillers.

The ideal filler is one that has a low risk of complications, is relatively predictable, and offers reproducible results. It would create a
natural appearance with minimal downtime and minimal side effects.
It would be easily tolerated by the patient with a low risk for allergic
reactions, eliminating the need for a skin test. It would be cost-
effective and provide a long-lasting but not permanent result.

WHAT DO SOFT TISSUE FILLER INJECTIONS ACCOMPLISH?

- The objective of using soft tissue fillers is to soften wrinkles,
  improve depressions, or add volume. These substances are used
  to fill in the fine or deep facial wrinkles, frown lines, smile
  lines, crow's feet, acne scars, and depressed traumatic scars
  (Figs. 16.1, 16.2). Some may also be used to enhance the lips
  by making them fuller. The only FDA-approved use of soft tissue fillers is in the treatment of facial soft tissue depressions.
  Consequently, enhancing the lips with these products is considered an off-label use.

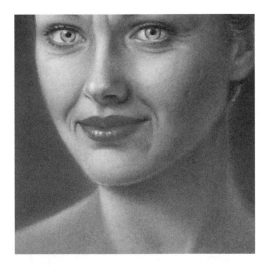

Figure 16.1. Over time, the loss of volume in our face results in prominent folds in the lower third of the face. Depressed scars are usually more noticeable than flat scars. (Courtesy American Society of Plastic Surgeons.)

- In adding volume to the soft tissues, the face becomes smoother and more youthful.
- With the exception of Sculptra Aesthetic, the results of these injections are immediate.

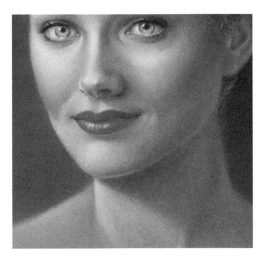

Figure 16.2. Soft tissue fillers may be used to soften the folds and depressions resulting from the loss of volume and natural aging. Some fillers may also be used to fill in depressed scars. (Courtesy American Society of Plastic Surgeons.)

- Since all of the FDA-approved fillers are metabolized by our body, their effect is temporary. They are absorbed over a period that can vary from three months to two years. The rate at which they are metabolized depends upon the nature of the filler used, the area into which it is injected, and the individual's response to the filler.

WHAT CAN I EXPECT DURING AND AFTER THE SOFT TISSUE FILLER INJECTION?

- All of the soft tissue filler treatments may be performed in an office setting, with you fully awake.
- Your face is cleansed, and the area to be injected is further treated with rubbing alcohol to minimize the potential for infection.
- The majority of these injections are performed with you in an upright position. Lying down or holding the head backward often diminishes the wrinkles and depressions in the face. Maintaining an upright position improves visualization of the areas to be treated and consequently allows more accurate placement of the filler.
- You may experience slight bleeding at the needle site; this is easily controlled with mild pressure.
- With the exception of Sculptra Aesthetic, you will see the effect of the soft tissue filler injections immediately.
- There is minimal recovery following the injections, and you may wear makeup shortly after the procedure.
- You may experience some redness for the first few hours at the injection site.
- You may also have swelling and bruising. These symptoms are more likely to occur and tend to last longer with the hyaluronic acid and Radiesse injections than with the collagen injections. The swelling tends to be more noticeable and potentially more intense with injections in the lips than anywhere else in the face.
- If you have a tendency to bruise, ice is helpful during and after the procedure.
- If you are undergoing any kind of injection procedures, you should try to avoid products that increase bleeding the week prior to your procedure, as these will increase the risk of bruising. A list of these products is found in the Appendix.

- Some individuals may develop "bumpy areas" where the soft tissue filler was injected. This may be a result of:

  - The filler being injected too superficially
  - Too much filler being placed in one area
  - Migration of the filler to one region—this is especially true of areas such as the lips and marionette lines
  - Inflammatory reaction to the injection

IS THERE TREATMENT FOR THE "BUMPY AREAS"?

- Massage is helpful to soften these bumps. If severe, a topical steroid cream or a small steroid injection may be attempted.
- If hyaluronic acid fillers are the cause of the bumps, a hyaluronidase product may be used to quickly dissolve them. This is considered an off-label use of hyaluronidase products.
- Often, however, only the body's natural metabolism of the injectable material over time will resolve the symptoms.

DO SOFT TISSUE FILLER INJECTIONS HURT?

- All injections are associated with pain. The discomfort associated with soft tissue filler injections is transient and typically does not last beyond the treatment session.
- The degree of discomfort is dependent upon the type of filler used and the area into which it is injected.
- There are three types of discomfort associated with soft tissue filler injections. The first is from the actual needle itself as it penetrates the skin. The second is due to the distension of the soft tissue as the filler is being injected. The third pain is due to the burning sensation of the substance itself.
- Collagen injections have a local anesthetic (Lidocaine) mixed with the collagen molecules and consequently are associated with only a slight degree of discomfort.
- If the hyaluronic acid fillers, Radiesse and Sculptra are not mixed with a local anesthetic prior to their injection into the soft tissues, they are associated with a greater degree of discomfort. Under these circumstances, the injections are more easily tolerated by using a topical anesthetic or by injecting a local anesthetic into the area being treated (similar to the technique used by dentists when working on teeth).

WHO IS NOT A CANDIDATE FOR SOFT TISSUE FILLER THERAPY?

- Patients with active inflammatory skin reactions, such as herpetic blisters, rashes, pimples, cysts, or hives, should postpone soft tissue filler injections until the condition has resolved.
- Patients with a strong history of herpetic blisters should undergo suppressive anti-herpetic treatment prior to undergoing soft tissue filler injections in the lips. However, this prophylactic treatment is considered an off-label use of anti-herpetic medications.
- Patients receiving immunosuppressive therapy should discuss obtaining soft tissue fillers with their physician to obtain clearance. At times, it is prudent to consider postponing these injections until patients are no longer receiving such treatment.
- Patients with connective tissue disorders may have increased susceptibility to hypersensitivity reactions, making soft tissue filler therapy unpredictable and perhaps imprudent. There is no data on the effect of these soft tissue fillers in this patient population.
- Women who are pregnant, attempting to become pregnant, or nursing should avoid soft tissue fillers since their safety during these conditions has not been established.
- The safety of soft tissue fillers has not been established in patients 12 years of age or younger.

ARE CERTAIN FILLERS MORE SUITABLE FOR CERTAIN CONDITIONS OR FOR CERTAIN PARTS OF THE FACE?

- Soft tissue fillers vary in terms of type, concentration, molecular weight, or degree of molecular cross linking.
- In general, fillers consisting of smaller molecules are more suitable for superficial lines and wrinkles, whereas those consisting of larger molecules are more appropriate for the deeper folds and wrinkles.

CAN DIFFERENT FILLERS BE USED TOGETHER IN ONE AREA?

- It has become common practice to use multiple fillers in the face. Certain fillers are more appropriate for different parts of the face than others.

- Under some circumstances, physicians may combine two fillers in the same region of the face. For example, they may place Radiesse along the deep plane of the nasolabial folds and layer Juvederm or Restylane above it, along a more superficial level.
- We do not have data on how well these fillers mix together once injected into the same region. However, to date, no adverse reactions have been reported.

COLLAGEN REPLACEMENT THERAPY

What Is Collagen?

- Collagen is a substance that is naturally found in many of our tissues, especially our skin. It is part of the skin's supporting structure. Over time, normal facial movements such as smiling, frowning, and talking lead to breakdown of collagen, thereby creating wrinkles, creases, and depressions. The timing of this process is influenced by time, genetics, and one's lifestyle. Sun exposure and smoking greatly contribute to collagen breakdown in the skin. Also, conditions such as acne scarring and traumatic injuries disturb the collagen deposition in the affected areas.
- Collagen may be injected back into these lines, creases, depressions, and scars to help soften their appearance.
- Although the use of injectable collagen has diminished due to the introduction of other soft tissue fillers, it is important to know the history of all of these products since clinical studies of newer soft tissue fillers often compare their effect to the effect of injectable collagen.
- There have been two major types of collagen replacement therapy available in the United States. These include bovine collagen and human collagen.

Bovine Collagen

- The original bovine collagen replacement therapy was available in three types:
  - Zyderm I
  - Zyderm II
  - Zyplast
- The three types varied in their concentration of collagen and the degree of cross-linking of the collagen molecules. The cross-linking

process is what makes a filler more robust and resistant to degradation.

- All three types of bovine collagen contained the local anesthetic Lidocaine for greater patient comfort.
  - ○ Zyderm I contained 35 mg/mL of non-cross-linked bovine collagen with Lidocaine.
  - ○ Zyderm II contained 65 mg/mL of non-cross-linked bovine collagen with Lidocaine.
  - ○ Zyplast contained 35 mg/mL of cross-linked bovine collagen with Lidocaine.
- Bovine collagen was harvested from a group of cows raised in the United States (Santa Barbara) specifically for the purpose of producing medical-grade injectable collagen.
- Bovine collagen replacement therapy had been tested extensively and had been proven safe and effective since 1976, and all three types of bovine collagen were approved for use by the Food and Drug Administration (FDA).

How Were Bovine Collagen Injections Done?

- For bovine collagen, two skin tests were required to check for possible allergic reactions and minimize the potential for development of an adverse response to the treatment. These two skin tests are not generally required for human collagen.

- The bovine collagen skin test included an injection of a small amount of collagen into the forearm. This was observed daily for a period of 30 days. The test screened for a preexisting allergy to bovine collagen. The area was monitored for evidence of redness, itching, swelling, soreness, and increasing firmness. If this test was negative, it was repeated once again after the initial 30-day period. Approximately 3 percent of the patients tested had a positive skin test, making them ineligible to receive bovine collagen treatment.

- The disadvantage of bovine collagen was the requirement of two negative skin tests prior to its use. Consequently, patients could not be treated at their first visit.

- If no positive reaction was noted following the two tests, then treatment was initiated. It should be understood that in spite of one or two negative skin tests, 1–2 percent of patients receiving bovine collagen treatment still demonstrated a reaction or a side effect that required further treatment.

- The bovine collagen lasted approximately two to three months, depending on the area into which it was injected and on the individual's unique response. Almost invariably, collagen injections in the lips lasted for a shorter period of time than injections in other parts of the face. Some patients metabolized bovine collagen faster than others. Consequently, some patients required injections only three or four times per year, while others required collagen replacement therapy more frequently.
- Since there was a need to wait two months for allergy test results prior to treatment, and there was potential for an allergic reaction even with two negative allergy tests, the use of bovine collagen became much more limited. Today, if a collagen product is required, most physicians will use human collagen. In view of this, the manufacturer (Allergan, Inc.) has discontinued the production of bovine collagen.

Human Collagen

- Human collagen replacement therapy is available in two types.
  - Cosmoderm
  - Cosmoplast
- These two forms of human collagen are derived from human foreskin. They are carefully processed to minimize the possibility of transmitting communicable diseases.
- Cosmoderm and Cosmoplast have been approved for use by the Food and Drug Administration (FDA) since March 2003.
- They do not require any form of skin testing.
- Cosmoderm and Cosmoplast both contain 35 mg/mL of human collagen and Lidocaine.
- Cosmoderm is comparable to Zyderm I in that it contains non-cross-linked collagen, making it ideal for superficial fine wrinkles.
- Cosmoplast is comparable to Zyplast in that it contains cross-linked collagen, making it suitable for lip enhancement and deep wrinkles.
- Similar to bovine collagen, Cosmoderm and Cosmoplast may be layered within the tissues to achieve optimal results.
- Cosmoplast and Cosmoderm injections are performed in the same manner as the bovine collagen injections, with the exception of not requiring a skin test.

HYALURONIC ACID

What Is a Hyaluronic Acid?

- Hyaluronic acid is a substance that is naturally found in all of our tissues.

- More than half of all of the hyaluronic acid in our body is found in our skin, where its ability to bind with water creates volume and allows the skin to remain well hydrated and supple.

- In addition to attracting water, hyaluronic acid also maintains the elasticity of the skin. Without hyaluronic acid, the skin would appear dry, withered, and wrinkled.

- The physiology, amount, and compartmentalization of hyaluronic acid change with age. These changes not only alter the hydration of the skin, but also decrease its elasticity, making it more susceptible to injury and infection.

- Hyaluronic acid provides structural support and elasticity to the skin. In large part, this is due to its ability to attract and bind water, thereby giving volume to the skin.

- Without hyaluronic acid, our skin would appear dry, withered, and wrinkled.

- As we age, there is a decrease in the levels of hyaluronic acid found in our skin. Consequently, the skin loses some of its volume and firmness, giving rise to wrinkles and folds.

- Hyaluronic acid gels, such as Restylane and Perlane (Medicis, Inc.), and Juvederm Ultra or Juvederm Ultra Plus (Allergan, Inc.), are manufactured in varying viscosities and are currently approved and distributed in Canada, Europe, and the United States.

- Hyaluronic derivatives are safe, are practical to use, and eliminate the need for allergy testing.

- Restylane, Perlane, Juvederm Ultra, and Juvederm Ultra Plus impart a natural texture and appearance to the skin.

- Although some of these products last longer than collagen, they are not permanent.

- Restylane, Perlane, Juvederm Ultra, and Juvederm Ultra Plus have the advantage of containing no animal components, and have been subjected to more extensive clinical evaluation than Hylaform, Hylaform Plus, or Captique.

- Despite similar properties, there are important differences between the different injectable hyaluronic acids. The main difference is the source of origin (avian or bacterial). Injectable hyaluronic acids may be obtained by either extraction from avian tissues (rooster combs) or a biotechnologic approach (bacterial source). Other significant differences include: the concentration of the hyaluronic acid; the individual particle size; whether the hyaluronic acid is cross-linked; the type of cross-linking agent used; the amount of cross-linking agent used; the gel viscosity; and the extent of studies available regarding safety, stability, and performance.

- Hyaluronic acids from an animal source (rooster combs) are not as commonly used as those from a bacterial source. They will be mentioned here for the sake of completion. After the roosters are sacrificed, their combs are finely minced and mixed with a solvent, and the hyaluronic acid is then extracted. These hyaluronic acids include:
  - Hylaform
  - Hylaform Plus
  - Captique
  - Prevelle Silk
- Non-animal (bacterial) hyaluronic acids are the current gold standard of injectable fillers. These include:
  - Restylane
  - Perlane
  - Juvederm Ultra
  - Juvederm Ultra Plus

What Is Restylane?

- Restylane is a crystal-clear-gel hyaluronic acid.
- It was developed in Uppsala, Sweden, in 1996.
- It has been used to treat wrinkles in over 60 counties throughout the world since 1996.
- Restylane was approved by the U.S. Food and Drug Administration (FDA) on December 12, 2003.
- Restylane is the first cosmetic dermal filler to be classified as a NASHA (Non-Animal Stabilized Hyaluronic Acid).
- Restylane is a sugar and is completely biocompatible. When metabolized, Restylane is broken down to water and carbon dioxide, both of which are naturally found in our body.

- Restylane has been the most studied hyaluronic acid worldwide.
- Restylane is available in three forms: Restylane, Restylane Fine Lines, and Perlane.
- Perlane was approved by the FDA in 2007. At this time, Restylane Fine Lines has not been approved for use in the United States.
- All Restylane preparations have a hyaluronic acid concentration of 20 mg/mL; however, the three preparations vary in the constituent particle size.
- Restylane Fine Lines, Restylane, and Perlane have particle sizes of 150 mm, 250 mm, and 1,000 mm, respectively. Smaller particle size is indicated for upper dermal injections, whereas the larger particles have increased lifting capacity and are indicated for mid- to deep-dermal areas.
- Restylane is produced by a streptococcus strain of bacteria. Because it is from a non-animal source, it is free of animal proteins. This limits the risk of transmission of animal diseases and allergic reactions. As such, Restylane does not typically require allergy testing.
- Restylane does have small traces of bacterial proteins and may induce a reaction in a very small percentage of the population. The incidence of adverse reactions to Restylane was reported to be 0.15 percent in 1999 and 0.06 percent in 2000. The decrease was due to using more purified material in the newer-generation of Restylane products.

What Is Juvederm Ultra?

- Juvederm Ultra is manufactured by Allergan, Inc., and is the result of more recent advances in hyaluronic acid research.
- Juvederm Ultra consists of cross-linked hyaluronic acid produced by *Streptococcus equi* bacteria and suspended in a physiologic buffer.
- It is formulated to a hyaluronic acid concentration of 24 or 30 mg/mL, based on the preparation.
- Juvederm Ultra has the highest hyaluronic acid concentration of all currently available hyaluronic acids.
- It comes in three different preparations, including: Juvederm 30, Juvederm 24HV (Juvederm Ultra), and Juvederm 30HV (Juvederm Ultra Plus). Juvederm Ultra and Juvederm Ultra Plus received FDA approval in the United States in June 2006.

- All other currently approved hyaluronic acid dermal fillers utilize a gel-particle suspension formulation. Unlike these, Juvederm Ultra and Juvederm Ultra Plus use *Hylacross Technology* (proprietary term), which results in a smooth gel formulation.

Where Can Hyaluronic Acids Be Injected in the Face?

- The FDA has approved hyaluronic acids for the treatment of moderate-to-severe facial wrinkles and folds, such as the nasolabial folds.
- Hyaluronic acids have been used cosmetically in areas of the face other than the nasolabial folds, but this is considered an off-label use. This means that hyaluronic acids are injected into areas of the face that extend beyond the areas initially described under FDA approval.
  - Areas of the face where hyaluronic acid use is considered off-label include:
    1. Lips
    2. Wrinkles around the lips
    3. Depressions along the tear trough ("dark circles under the eyes")
    4. Deep wrinkles or furrows in between the eyebrows
    5. Depressed scars
    6. Hollowness or depressions within the cheeks

How Long Do the Effects of Hyaluronic Acids Last?

- The longevity of the injected soft tissue fillers depends on the filler used, the area into which it is injected and on the individual's unique response.
- In general, treatment with Perlane will last longer than treatment with Restylane and treatment with Juvederm Ultra Plus will last longer than treatment with Juvederm Ultra.
- Soft tissue fillers are metabolized faster in areas where there is significant movement and last longer in areas with very little movement. For example, the same filler may last six months in the nasolabial folds, and nine months along the tear trough, but only four months in the lips.
- It is important to remember that each person may have a slightly different reaction to one filler relative to another. In some, Juvederm Ultra will last longer that Restylane, while in others, Restylane will

last longer. Under your doctor's recommendations, it is best for you to use the products that best agree with your desired goals. If the hyaluronic acid that you are using is not lasting long enough or is easily palpable, consider trying one of the others in effort to see if you will have a better response.

NON-HYALURONIC ACID INJECTABLE SOFT TISSUE FILLERS

What Is Radiesse?

- Radiesse consists of calcium-based microspheres suspended in a water-based gel.
- Once injected into the skin, it stimulates the formation of your own collagen. The calcium is thought to provide a scaffold to support and stimulate this process of collagen formation.
- Radiesse is injected into facial depressions to help restore volume and temporarily fill in the folds.
- A popular but off-label use of Radiesse is enhancement of the midface. In this technique, Radiesse is injected directly over the cheekbones in effort to augment them and improve their contour. This treats the flatness along the anterior cheeks that develops with age and often causes the face to appear drawn.
- Radiesse is thought to last approximately one year in the majority of patients, but individual results may vary.

What Is Sculptra Aesthetic?

- Sculptra Aesthetic contains primarily Poly-L-Lactic acid, a bio-compatible synthetic product found in dissolvable suture material.
- It has been used cosmetically in Europe since 1999 and received FDA approval for cosmetic use in the United States in 2009.
- It is indicated for the correction of shallow to deep nasolabial folds, contour deficiencies, and facial wrinkles.
- It enhances the tissues by stimulating collagen formation.
- It works differently from the other soft tissue fillers. The effect of Sculptra Aesthetic is not immediate. The process is gradual and usually requires three injection sessions over a few months.
- Sculptra Aesthetic cannot be injected into or near muscles, since it may lead to a foreign body reaction (firm areas of product and scar tissue) formation. Consequently, it cannot be used in the lips.

- Sculptra Aesthetic is thought to last approximately two years in the majority of patients.

What Is a Fat Transfer Procedure?

- This involves the use of one's own fat in order to fill in depressions or add volume to the face.
- The fat is usually harvested from an area such as the abdomen, the buttocks, or the inner part of the knees.
- It is then immediately processed to remove blood, blood products, fluid, and disrupted fat cells. The healthy fat cells are saved for use.
- The healthy fat cells are then immediately injected into the facial area in need of volume to restore a more youthful appearance.
- Fresh fat has the best chance of establishing a blood supply in the facial area into which it is injected. Establishing a healthy blood supply allows the fat to survive, thereby providing long-term correction.
- The advantages of fat transfer are twofold:
  - We cannot be allergic to it. It is easily tolerated by our body because it is our own tissue.
  - Some of the injected fat will establish a healthy blood supply and survive long term.
- The disadvantages of fat transfer are also twofold:
  - Fat is unpredictable in terms of its survival, as it may not establish a healthy blood supply in its new location. Consequently, some of it will dissipate. Since the percentage of fat survival is unpredictable, the appropriate amount of overcorrection in an attempt to compensate for the partial survival cannot be exact.
  - There is more involved with harvesting and preparing fat than there is with using one of the other FDA-approved soft tissue fillers. The fat must be removed from one area of the body. This harvesting may be performed under local anesthesia, with you fully awake if only a small amount of fat is needed, or with sedation if larger amounts of fat are needed. The area is usually tender and bruised during the healing process. The extensiveness of recovery depends on the amount of fat harvested and the area from which it is removed. The fat must then be processed to remove any blood products, disrupted fat cells, and fluid. This is usually accomplished by spinning the harvested fat in a centrifuge to separate it into its various constituents. The unwanted products are then decanted, and the desired fat cells are placed into syringes for immediate injection.

Aesthetic Breast Surgery

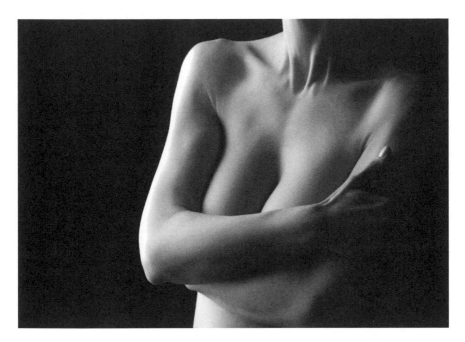

Stuart Rogers Photography

17

Breast Augmentation (Augmentation Mammaplasty)

WHAT IS A BREAST AUGMENTATION, AND WHAT DOES IT ACCOMPLISH?

- It involves placement of saline-filled or silicone-filled implants behind the breast tissue or behind the chest muscles.
- It enhances the body contour for women who feel that their breasts are too small (Fig. 17.1).
- It may correct the changes in breast volume and shape after pregnancy or after weight loss.
- It may be used as a reconstructive technique following certain types of breast surgery.
- In some cases of breast asymmetry or poor development, breast implants may be used to help achieve improved symmetry.
- There are six questions to be answered when undergoing a breast augmentation:
  - Is there a need for a breast lift as well, or is this strictly a breast augmentation?
  - What type of implant will be used—saline or silicone?
  - Where will the incision be placed?
  - Will the implant be placed above or below the muscle?
  - What shape of implant is most appropriate?
  - What size of implant is most appropriate or desirable?

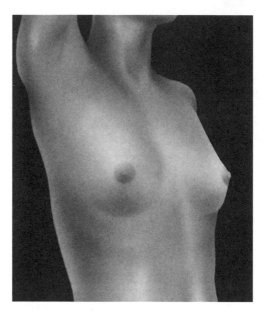

Figure 17.1.   Breast augmentation is usually done to balance a difference in breast size, to improve body contour, or as a reconstructive technique following surgery. (Courtesy American Society of Plastic Surgeons.)

HOW IS IT DONE?

- There are four skin incisions possible for placement of breast implants: along the lower portion of the areola (colored skin around the nipple); under the breast within the natural crease; in the axilla (underarm); and through the navel (Fig. 17.2). The navel incision is not commonly used.
- Once the incision is made through the skin, it is continued through the breast tissue until the surface of the chest muscle is identified.
- The pocket is then created for the implant, either above (subglandular) the pectoralis major muscle or behind (submuscular) the pectoralis major muscle (Fig. 17.3).
- If placed above the pectoralis major muscle, the implant is placed behind the breast tissue. The implant is not placed within the breast tissue.
- In the majority of patients, the pocket must be advanced towards the center to create better cleavage. In some cases, the pocket needs to be advanced below the natural breast crease to allow a more natural position of the implant after the healing process.

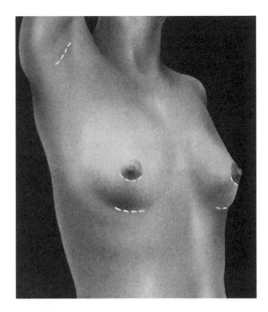

Figure 17.2. Incisions are made to keep scars as inconspicuous as possible, in the breast crease, around the nipple, or in the crease under the arm. Breast tissue and skin are lifted to create a pocket for each implant. (Courtesy American Society of Plastic Surgeons.)

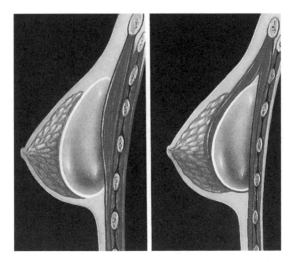

Figure 17.3. The breast implant may be inserted directly under the breast tissue or beneath the chest wall muscle. (Courtesy American Society of Plastic Surgeons.)

Failure to take these steps into consideration may lead to widely displaced implants and/or high-sitting implants.

• Different shapes of the implants are currently used depending upon the individual patient's needs. Women will have far more options for breast implant shape over the next few years. There are implants being evaluated that will provide a nearly customized implant shape based on the patient's needs. These implants will vary in their height, width, and projection. Once they are FDA approved, they will allow plastic surgeons and patients to have greater options. Whether these implants will provide an added long-term benefit that will justify the greater expense and potentially the larger incisions remains to be seen.

• Although the two breast implant manufacturers in the United States may use slightly different terminology, the currently available FDA-approved implant shapes include:

○ Round

1. Low profile
2. Moderate profile
3. High profile

○ Tear-shaped (also called "anatomical" or "contoured")

1. Moderate profile
2. High profile

HOW DOES ONE DECIDE WHICH SHAPE IMPLANT IS MOST APPROPRIATE?

• The width and diameter of the chest, the width of the breast, and the desired future size of the breasts play a critical role in choosing the profile of the implant.

• In thin patients with a narrow chest who desire a full breast, the high-profile implant may provide the desired size without too much fullness along the sides of the breast.

• In patients with an average or wide chest, a moderate profile implant provides the desired size with a greater chance of achieving the desired degree of cleavage.

• The roles of the round or tear-shaped implants are less clearly defined and depend on the patient's anatomy and surgeon's preference.

- It is important to clarify that patients will *not* have breasts that look "round" if the surgeon uses a round implant.
- Tear-shaped implants may not necessarily look more natural, especially if they shift clockwise or counterclockwise. All tear-shaped implants are textured. This allows them to adhere to the patient's tissues and minimizes the chance of rotating or flipping.

HOW DOES ONE DECIDE WHETHER TO PLACE THE IMPLANT BEHIND THE PECTORALIS MAJOR MUSCLE (SUBMUSCULAR) OR BEHIND THE BREAST TISSUE (SUBGLANDULAR)?

- In the majority of patients, it is recommended that implants be placed behind the chest muscle.
- Advantages of placing implants behind the chest muscles include:
  - Less interference with future mammograms
  - Less potential of capsular contracture
  - Greater coverage of the implant by the patient's own tissue, thereby decreasing the chance of visible rippling along the upper pole of the breast (especially important in thin women)
  - A more natural and youthful slope to the breast as it projects from the chest
  - A greater chance of maintaining the desired position of the implant in the future
- Role for placement of implants in front of the chest muscle
  - When a woman presents after having lost a significant amount of breast tissue either following childbirth and breast-feeding, or following significant weight loss, or if she simply developed droopy breasts during adolescence, it is a very different patient from the woman who presents with very small breasts that never developed to any substantial degree.
  - Women who have always had small breasts that did not droop do not have the issue of excess skin. The decision to place the implant behind the muscle in these patients is associated with an aesthetically pleasing result.
  - In women who have excess skin or drooping of the breast, placing the implant behind the muscle almost always necessitates a breast lift. Breast lifts are associated with scars that can vary from minor to extensive, depending on the degree of lifting necessary.
  - Women who fall in this category and are unwilling to accept the scars associated with a breast lift need to consider not having the breast augmentation altogether. In some cases, such as those with only a

slight amount of drooping and a fair amount of breast tissue, the implants may be placed in front of the chest muscle. This allows the implant to fill out the skin envelope and corrects the slight deflation that has occurred in the breasts without the need for a formal breast lift. This is not recommended when a women has significant drooping or a significant amount of excess skin. It is not wise to use a very large implant to fill out the excess tissue hoping it will lift the breast. When there is significant drooping, the patient requires a breast lift.

   o When large implants are placed in front of the chest muscle in hopes of filling out the excess skin, it potentially leads to additional complications. Often, using large implants for this purpose will increase the sagging and make the future breast lift surgery more challenging. Furthermore, it may create a very unnatural and undesirable shape to the breast.

WHEN ARE THE SUTURES REMOVED FOLLOWING A BREAST AUGMENTATION?

- Most plastic surgeons use dissolvable sutures.
- If non-dissolvable sutures are used, usually these are removed after one week.

ARE THERE ANY SCARS WITH BREAST AUGMENTATION?

- Whenever an incision is made in the human face or body, it heals with a scar. All of the incisions used for breast augmentation surgery are very small, measuring approximately 2–3 cm (saline) or 4.5–6 cm (silicone) in length. They are usually not prominent once completely healed (Fig. 17.4).

WHAT KIND OF ANESTHESIA IS RECOMMENDED DURING A BREAST AUGMENTATION?

- The procedure may be performed using either general or twilight anesthesia.
- When implants are being placed behind the chest muscle, most surgeons recommend general anesthesia.

IS THERE A GREAT DEAL OF PAIN WITH BREAST AUGMENTATION?

- Most of the pain is experienced during the first 48 hours. Patients describe it as a pressure-type pain and tightness.

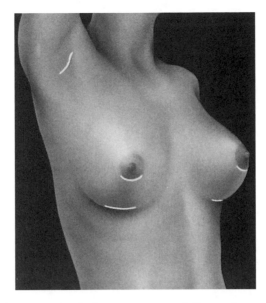

Figure 17.4. After surgery, the breasts appear fuller and more natural in tone and contour. The scars fade with time. (Courtesy American Society of Plastic Surgeons.)

- Implants placed behind the chest muscle are associated with greater pain than those placed in front of the chest muscle.
- Many plastic surgeons use a device called the "pain pump." This delivers a local anesthetic to each breast through a very thin tube during the first 48 hours after surgery.
- Despite the pain pump, most patients will require additional pain medication.
- If the implants are placed behind the muscle, there is the potential for muscle spasm, and a muscle relaxant such as Valium is also helpful.

WHAT IS THE RECOVERY TIME FOLLOWING BREAST AUGMENTATION?

- It will take approximately one week before patients are feeling relatively well again.
- Implants placed behind the muscle are associated with a longer recovery.

- In cases in which the implants are placed behind the muscle, limited use of the arms helps in keeping the pain under control.

WHO NEEDS A MAMMOGRAM BEFORE BREAST AUGMENTATION SURGERY?

- Women who are ages 35–40 and have never had a mammogram
- Women over the age of 40 and who have not had a mammogram within the year prior to the breast augmentation
- Women of any age who have had an abnormal mammogram or a family history of breast cancer
- Women of any age who have abnormal findings on a breast examination

DO BREAST IMPLANTS INCREASE THE RISK OF BREAST CANCER?

- No. There has never been any data to suggest that having saline or silicone breast implants is associated with an increased risk of breast cancer.

WHAT CAN I EXPECT AFTER BREAST IMPLANT SURGERY?

- When you awaken in the recovery room following breast augmentation, you will have a dressing wrapped around your chest. This is intended to provide slight compression and adequate support. Some surgeons also use a band across the upper pole of the breasts to help minimize upward migration of the implants during the immediate period after surgery. This band is more likely to be used when the implants are placed behind the muscle.
- The pain is typically described as a pressure and tightness across the chest. You will find that much of the pain will subside after the first 48 hours following surgery.
- If a "pain pump" is used, it will be removed by your surgeon after the first 24–48 hours.
- Expect to have a slight burning sensation along the incisions. This is easily treated with the prescribed pain medication.

- If the implants are placed behind the chest muscles:
  - The recovery is slightly longer than when they are placed in front of the chest muscles.
  - You may experience muscle spasms, and the prescribed muscle relaxants are helpful.
  - During the first 24 hours, you may feel somewhat limited raising your arms. However, you will be able to attend to basic needs, such as eating, brushing your teeth, and simple hygiene.
  - After the first two to three days, you will begin to feel comfortable using your arms for activities of daily living, such as showering, combing your hair, and getting dressed.
  - When the dressings are removed after the first 24–48 hours, the implants are typically sitting higher than they will be eventually after they take their final position. This may be a source of anxiety unless you are aware of the implants' normal tendency toward upward migration during the early healing phase.
- You can expect to have some bruising and be slightly swollen for the first two weeks.
- Although rare, some surgeons consider the use of drains after a breast augmentation. In these circumstances, a very small drain is placed within each breast to help remove any blood or serum from around the implant. These drains are thought to decrease bruising and potentially capsular contracture. If used, they are removed by your surgeon within the first 24–48 hours following surgery.
- You may feel numbness or increased sensitivity in the nipple area. In the majority of cases, this is temporary and will subside over a period of weeks to months.
- You will have some swelling after surgery. The swelling will significantly decrease over the first two to four weeks. When swelling occurs, one breast may appear larger or higher than the other. Be patient. As the swelling subsides, the breasts will take their final shape and appear more natural.
- Although the implants drop significantly by three months, it may take up to one year before they take their final position. The changes that occur after the first three months are subtle in nature and noticeable by you and by your physician, but not usually by others.
- Once the swelling subsides, you may feel rippling along the lower outer pole of each breast. Even when the implants are placed behind the muscle, the outer lower segment of each implant is not usually covered by muscle. The pectoralis major

muscle does not extend far enough to cover the entire lower outer pole of the implant. The rippling is more noticeable in thinner individuals, since there is less tissue coverage over the implant. Although there is less rippling with silicone implants than there is with saline implants, thin women should expect to have some rippling with either type of implant due to insufficient tissue coverage.

- Over the course of months to years, your implants may shift outward, downward, or upward. They may rupture or become firm (capsular contracture). Your own tissue may sag over the implants, giving an unnatural appearance to the breasts. Depending on their degree, these changes may necessitate additional surgery. The most common cause of re-operation in the first five years after breast augmentation is capsular contracture.

WHAT IS CAPSULAR CONTRACURE?

- Capsular contracture is the result of excessive scar tissue that forms around the breast implant. Although every patient will form scar tissue around their breast implants, the quality and extent of scar tissue vary greatly between patients and can even vary between the two breast in the same patient.

- In the majority of cases, the scar is soft and does not impact the shape or softness of the implant. However, in cases in which the scar thickens, it begins to tighten around the implant. The degree of tightening affects the degree of capsular contracture.

- The Baker classification of capsular contracture is used to describe the degree of capsular contracture. There are four grades:

  o Baker Grade I is a natural soft breast
  o Baker Grade II is a breast that is firm
  o Baker Grade III is a breast that is firm with visible distortion
  o Baker Grade IV is a breast that is firm, distorted and painful

- The etiology of capsular contracture is not completely understood. In general, the potential for capsular contracture is unpredictable in patients who are undergoing breast augmentation for the first time. Although we know that there are certain conditions that may increase or decrease the incidence of capsular contracture, we do not know enough to prevent it.

- Capsular contracture can occur with saline or silicone implants.
- Placing the implants behind the pectoralis major muscle has been associated with a lower rate of capsular contracture. The movement of the muscle is thought to massage the implant, thereby decreasing the likelihood of thick scar tissue to form.
- An infection or bleeding around the breast implant has been associated with a higher rate of capsular contracture.
- Patients who have had problems with capsular contracture with their initial breast augmentation are more likely to have similar problems following subsequent breast augmentation procedures.

WHAT ARE SOME OF THE OTHER POTENTIAL COMPLICATIONS OF BREAST AUGMENTATION?

- Implants may shift over time. This may lead to the implants sitting too far apart or falling below their ideal position. When they fall below the level of the breast tissue, the condition is referred to as "bottoming out" and requires surgical correction.
- Although more rare, the implants may shift towards the center of the chest, obliterating the natural cleavage plane between the breasts. This condition is referred to as "synmastia" or "symmastia." It is more likely to occur if very large implants are used relative to what the patient's tissue can handle, or if the patient has a depression along the central aspect of her rib cage, or if the tissue is dissected too far towards the midline during the initial surgery. This is more difficult to fix surgically than the other types of implant malposition.

HOW DO I CARE FOR MYSELF AFTER BREAST AUGMENTATION SURGERY?

- It is important that you take the prescribed antibiotics to help prevent infection.
- You should use the pain medication and muscle relaxants as prescribed in order to feel comfortable, but not overly sedated.
- You may shower as soon as the original dressings used in surgery and pain pump (if used) are removed. Usually, these are removed by your surgeon 24–48 hours after surgery. You should take showers and avoid baths during the first four weeks. Shower water is

considered clean, but bath water is not. Exposing your fresh incisions to unclean water may predispose you to an infection. After four weeks, the incisions are healed sufficiently to expose them to bath water without much risk.

- If your implants are placed behind the muscle, expect that raising your arms will be uncomfortable at first.

  o Use your arms only for activities of daily living during the first two weeks.

  o You should avoid heavy lifting or overhead arm activities for four to six weeks.

  o You should avoid chest exercises, as well as aerobic arm activity that works the chest muscles, for six weeks.

  o You should avoid driving until you are comfortable moving your arms and are no longer taking pain medication.

  o You may return to work when comfortable and not prohibited by the degree of activity required by your occupation. For patients returning to office duties, usually the recovery time is three to five days when implants are placed above the muscle, and five to seven days when implants are placed behind the muscle. For professions requiring a great deal of lifting or other intense physical activity, a longer recovery time is needed.

- You should not wear underwire bras until the implants have dropped into their desired position. Your plastic surgeon may advise you to wear a sports bra or a bra without an underwire during this initial period, depending upon your individual situation. Under these circumstances, he or she will determine when you are ready to wear a regular bra.

- Some plastic surgeons advise their patients to wear a compression band over the upper pole of the breast to help the implants settle into place. This band should be worn at all times, except when showering, until your surgeon informs you to discontinue its use.

- The two most significant (and fortunately, rare) complications during the first two weeks following breast augmentation surgery are internal bleeding and infection. If bleeding occurs, it is very rare to have it occur on both sides. The asymmetry in symptoms is very important in defining the situation. Your surgeon must be notified immediately if any of the following nine symptoms occur:

  o Signs of internal bleeding:

    1. Significant asymmetrical swelling
    2. Excessive asymmetrical pain
    3. Sudden increase in the degree of bruising

o Signs of infection:

1. Spreading redness along one or both breasts
2. A foul odor along the incision
3. Drainage or pus from the incision site
4. Excessive warmth along the breast
5. Excessive localized tenderness
6. Fever

- If there is significant bleeding (hematoma), it is a surgical emergency.
- If there is an infection of the implant, it requires removal of the implant until there is adequate healing of the tissues. Usually this is over a period of several weeks and may be as long as three months.
- If your implants are behind the muscle, you are massaging them every time that you move your arms. If they are in front of the muscle, it is important to massage them regularly. Massaging the implants is believed to decrease the chance of capsular contracture. The timing of when to begin massage depends on the tenderness of the breasts, the extent of bruising, the extent of swelling, and your surgeon's preference. It is important to begin massage as soon as your surgeon advises you to do so. If your implants are above the muscle, you should try to massage them daily during the first several months following your procedure.

  o Different surgeons advise different massaging techniques. The goal is to move the implants so as to minimize the potential of thick scar tissue from forming around them.

  o Although there are many techniques, my preferred approach is the following:

  1. Step 1: Push the breasts toward midline, attempting to have them touch, and hold for a count of 10. Repeat 10 times.
  2. Step 2: Pace both hands along the upper pole of each breast and push directly towards your back. Hold for a count of 10. Repeat 10 times. This movement helps the implants fall into the desired position faster. If the implants are already at their desired level (not too high), you do not need to do this step.
  3. You should try to perform the above exercises several times daily.

- Breast evaluation following breast augmentation surgery

  o You must continue monthly self–breast exams following breast augmentation surgery. It is important for you to learn how to examine your breasts and differentiate the implant from your own tissue.

Once the majority of the swelling has subsided (approximately three to six months), the examination becomes much easier to perform.

o You should obtain your mammograms in a medical center experienced with performing and interpreting mammograms of patients with breast implants. The Ecklund mammogram technique is recommended in breast implant patients. This involves pulling the breast tissue forward while pushing the breast implant back, in order to allow improved visualization of the breast tissue.

o A mammogram is usually recommended approximately 6–12 months after surgery to establish a new baseline for later reference. You should check with your plastic surgeon as to the exact timing of your first mammogram following surgery.

o Patients should continue undergoing mammograms according to the following schedule unless otherwise dictated by their physician or family history:

1. Age 35–40: Screening mammogram
2. Over age 40: Mammogram once a year

HOW LONG WILL THE BREAST IMPLANTS LAST?

- Breast implants are not lifetime devices. In general, the currently available saline and silicone breast implants are given a life span of 10 years. However, some may rupture earlier, and some may last much longer.

- The risk of rupture is approximately 2 percent per implant per year. The older the implant, the greater the likelihood of rupture.

- The diagnosis of saline implant rupture is easily made on physical exam. In fact, it is usually made by the patient who notes a decrease in the size of one breast. The diagnosis of silicone implant rupture is much more difficult, since there may be no evidence of a change in breast size. Studies have shown that even plastic surgeons experienced in breast augmentation will diagnose a rupture on physical examination only 30 percent of the time. Consequently, the FDA recommends that women who have silicone breast implants undergo an MRI evaluation to rule out implant rupture every two years, starting three years following their surgery.

- Both Allergan, Inc. and Mentor have FDA-approved saline and silicone breast implants. Both companies provide patients with a five-year warranty against implant rupture and the ability to purchase an extended warranty for an additional five years. Since the risk of rupture increases with the age of the implant, most surgeons recommend that patients obtain the additional warranty.

ARE THERE ALTERNATIVES TO BREAST IMPLANT SURGERY TO INCREASE BREAST SIZE?

- Although some physicians have recommended the use of devices such as the Brava System, and there are advertisements promoting the use of "herbal supplements," the long-term effectiveness and potential risks of such methods have not been fully established.

- Some plastic surgeons perform fat injections in the breasts to enhance breast size. These procedures must be performed by surgeons experienced in fat grafting techniques. Simply injecting large amounts of fat into the breast may result in firm areas of "fat necrosis." These are collections of fat that never established a healthy blood supply. As such, the fat dies and forms a firm tissue that may be mistaken for a suspicious lump. When performed well, fat grafting technique may be used to perform a modest breast augmentation. It may take a woman from an A to a B breast cup size, but it is not recommended for a more significant increase.

WHEN IS IT THE RIGHT TIME FOR BREAST IMPLANT SURGERY?

- The majority of patients usually present for a breast augmentation at two points in life. The first group is women in their 20s or 30s prior to having children and the second group is women in their 40s or early 50s after they have completed having children and need to deal with all of the changes that occurred due to childbearing.

- Younger patients may be good candidates for the procedure, depending upon their physical, psychological, and emotional maturity.

- Older patients may be good candidates for the procedure depending upon their health status. Patients in this group may need more than a simple augmentation; often, they may need a breast lift as well. The different techniques of breast lifting will be discussed under their own chapter.

18

Breast Reduction
(Reduction Mammaplasty)

WHAT IS A BREAST REDUCTION, AND WHAT DOES IT ACCOMPLISH?

- This procedure is used to treat a condition known as *mammary hypertrophy*, which describes disproportionately large and heavy breasts (Fig. 18.1).
- The breast is a complex combination of breast gland (milk-producing) tissue, fat, and skin. Breast size is affected by puberty, pregnancy, menopause, and weight. A breast reduction involves the removal of some of the breast tissue (gland and fat), a segment of the areola (brown area around the nipple), and a portion of the skin from the breasts in order to reduce their size and place them into a more uplifted position.
- It reduces the overall size of the breasts, the size of enlarged areolas (pink/brown area around the nipple), and the fullness along the sides of the chest if this is due to excess breast tissue.
- It lifts the breasts to a more youthful position.
- It permits easier breast examinations and reduces the discomfort or restriction of activity due to heavy breasts.

WHO ARE GOOD CANDIDATES FOR A BREAST REDUCTION?

- Women with large breasts who experience any of the following conditions may be good candidates for this procedure:
  - Back, shoulder, and neck pain due to the excess weight of the breasts.
  - Difficulty maintaining good posture due to breast size.

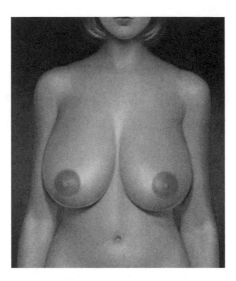

Figure 18.1.   Heavy breasts can lead to physical discomfort, shoulder indentations due to tight bra straps, and extreme self-consciousness. (Courtesy American Society of Plastic Surgeons.)

- o Painful shoulder grooving from bra strap indentations due to heaviness of the breasts.
- o Limited exercise tolerance due to breast weight.
- o Skin irritation under the breasts due to constant rubbing/sweating of the breasts over the underlying skin.
- o Difficulty performing adequate self–breast examinations for cancer detection due to breast size.

HOW IS A BREAST REDUCTION PERFORMED?

- • Techniques vary tremendously but follow basic rules.
- • The most common procedure is the "pedicle" approach, which allows the nipple to remain attached to the breast tissue at all times.
- • The most common type of incision is a keyhole-shaped incision that encircles the areola, then extends down along the midline of the breast, then extends to follow the natural crease of the fold underneath the breast (Fig. 18.2). There are no incisions along the upper pole of the breast.

  - o The extra fat, skin, and breast tissue are removed.
  - o The nipple and areola are then moved upward to their more youthful and higher position (Fig. 18.3).

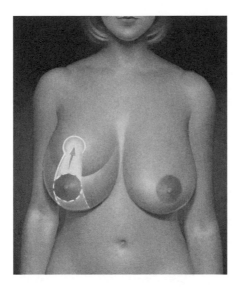

Figure 18.2. Incisions for a breast reduction outline the area of skin, breast tissue, and fat to be removed and designate the new position for the nipple. (Courtesy American Society of Plastic Surgeons.)

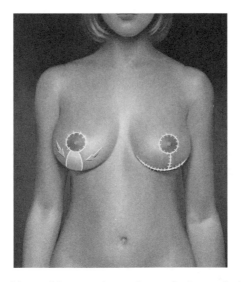

Figure 18.3. The skin and breast tissue formerly located above and around the nipple are brought together to reshape the breast. Sutures close the incisions, giving the breast its new contour. (Courtesy American Society of Plastic Surgeons.)

- In cases in which the breasts are extremely large and sagging, some surgeons may recommend a technique called "free nipple graft," in which the nipple and areola are temporarily removed during the surgery until the reduction is complete and then placed in their desired position at the end of the surgery. This procedure is rarely necessary. The majority of even extremely large reductions may be performed with the pedicle approach described above.

WHERE ARE THE SCARS FOLLOWING A BREAST REDUCTION?

- Typically the scars are around the areola, down the center of the breast, and along the crease underneath the breast (Fig. 18.4). The length of the scars along the breast crease depends on the type of technique used and the size of the reduction necessary. In general, larger reductions require longer crease scars.
- Every attempt is made to decrease the width and length of the breast reduction scars. Some surgeons perform small and moderate breast reductions using incisions that result in a circular scar around the areola and a vertical scar along the center of the breast without a scar along the breast crease. Often, this is referred to as "lollipop" incision. In these situations, the final shape of the breast

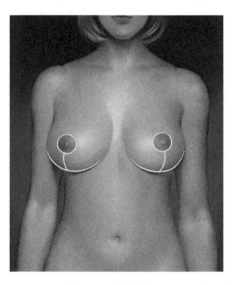

Figure 18.4. The scars around the areola, below it, and in the crease under the breast are permanent, but generally fade over time. (Courtesy American Society of Plastic Surgeons.)

may not be apparent immediately after surgery. There may be a slight bunching of the tissue along the vertical incision that corrects itself over time. This is especially true when larger breast reductions are performed through this short scar technique.

- The scars are initially red in everyone. In individuals with fair skin tones, they fade to pink and later to white. In individuals with darker skin tones, they may become slightly brown before they fade. All of these changes occur over the course of one to three years. It is important to protect the scars from sun exposure during this period, as sun exposure will often cause the scars to become darker in most individuals.

- The scars along the crease under the breast are usually the ones to become slightly raised or widened. The remaining scars usually heal very well.

- The final shape of the breasts may not be completely evident until one year after surgery. Initially, the breasts may appear "boxy." This is more likely to be true of larger reductions. However, the breasts usually round out nicely and take on a more natural shape over the subsequent 6–12 months.

WHAT TYPE OF ANESTHESIA IS RECOMMENDED DURING A BREAST REDUCTION?

- Typically, most breast reductions are performed under general anesthesia.

HOW LONG IS THE RECOVERY TIME?

- It will take approximately one week before you are feeling relatively well again.
- Most patients are able to return to activities of daily living, such as personal grooming, within the first two days.
- For women with physically strenuous jobs, most surgeons recommend a two-week period of recovery.

IS BREAST REDUCTION SURGERY A PAINFUL PROCEDURE?

- Most women report a very mild pain that is easily controlled with the prescribed pain medication.
- The majority of the pain resolves after the first two days.

ARE THERE ANY ALTERNATIVES TO A BREAST REDUCTION?

- In cases in which the breasts are only minimally enlarged, the woman should weigh the potential benefit of a small breast reduction against the potential scars and risks of the procedure. In these cases, she may elect not to undergo surgery. Support garments may be helpful, even though they do not correct the basic underlying condition.
- Weight reduction will reduce the fatty component of the breast but not affect the glandular tissue, which is approximately 50 percent of the overall breast volume. Similarly, liposuction removes fat but not glandular tissue. Nonetheless, women who are significantly overweight should try weight reduction prior to undergoing surgery. Not only will they be in better physical condition to undergo surgery, but also when they are closer to their ideal weight, they will be in a better position to determine whether or not they truly need a breast reduction.

ARE THERE ANY POTENTIAL ADVERSE EFFECTS TO NOT UNDERGOING A BREAST REDUCTION?

- Excess weight along the chest for years may affect your posture and cause back, shoulder, and neck pain.
- Excessive weight on the bra straps may cause painful shoulder grooving.
- With normal aging, the breast weight may become increasingly more difficult to tolerate and limit your activity level.
- Sagging heavy breasts may produce skin irritation along the folds of the breasts. Over time, this may lead to discoloration of the skin along the folds.
- Large breasts may make it difficult for you to perform adequate self–breast examinations for cancer detection.

WHAT ARE THE LIMITATIONS OF A BREAST REDUCTION?

- Breast reductions cannot reduce breast size without obvious scars.
- All humans are asymmetrical. You should not expect perfect symmetry from this procedure.

- Breast reduction surgery will not eliminate all of your stretch marks.
- If you have very wide breasts with breast tissue extending under the arms towards the back, a breast reduction may leave the breasts somewhat boxy. Once the breasts have healed and their final shape has been determined (over the course 6–12 months), the excess tissue along the sides of the breasts extending towards the back may be addressed using liposuction.

HOW LONG WILL THE EFFECTS OF A BREAST REDUCTION LAST?

- Although breast tissue has been permanently removed, subsequent breast sagging may occur as the result of aging, loss of skin elasticity, and the effect of gravity on the remaining breast tissue.
- The future size of the breasts is also influenced by weight gain or loss, pregnancy, and menopause.
- Re-development and enlargement of breast tissue following breast reduction has been reported, but it is extremely uncommon. If a breast reduction is performed in an adolescent girl prior to completion of puberty, there is a potential that her breasts will continue to grow after surgery until she has completed puberty. Also, if a breast reduction patient gains or loses a considerable amount of weight, it will impact the size and shape of her new breasts.

IS THERE ANY EFFECT ON THE INCIDENCE OF BREAST CANCER FOLLOWING A BREAST REDUCTION?

- There is no increase in the incidence of breast cancer after breast reduction.
- As with all women, there is a need for lifelong follow up for cancer detection.
- Mammograms may be recommended prior to surgery to determine if there are any suspicious areas present that should undergo biopsy prior to or during surgery.
- Mammograms are usually recommended approximately 6–12 months after surgery to establish a new baseline for later reference.

- After surgery, patients should continue undergoing mammograms according to the following schedule unless otherwise dictated by their physician or family history:

  ○ Age 35-40: Screening mammogram
  ○ Over age 40: Mammogram once a year

WHEN ARE THE SUTURES REMOVED?

- Most surgeons use sutures that are buried under the skin and are dissolvable.
- Some surgeons will use sutures that require removal. In these situations, the sutures are removed during the first two to four weeks following surgery.
- The third type of suture is a non-dissolvable suture that stays under the skin for many months after surgery. This is not visible to the patient, but serves the function of keeping tension off of the incisions to allow a finer scar.
- Since there are many types of surgical preferences for closing the incisions, every surgeon will advise the patient of what technique he or she prefers.

WHAT CAN I EXPECT AFTER BREAST REDUCTION SURGERY?

- When you awaken in the recovery room, you will have a compression dressing around the chest. This will consist of gauze and Ace wraps, or possibly a surgical brassiere.
- There will be a drainage tube placed within each breast to drain the excess fluid for the first 24–72 hours. All incisions will be covered with surgical tape to further protect them.
- Most patients report a stinging-type pain along both breasts. The pain is not severe in nature. Women describe it as moderate during the first day, diminishing to a very mild tenderness over the subsequent two days. Most of the pain is easily tolerated with the prescribed pain medication.
- You can expect to have bruising and swelling. The bruising will be visibly worse at 48 hours after surgery than immediately after the procedure. It may gravitate downward along the rib cage. You can expect it to diminish over the subsequent two weeks.

- The skin of the breasts and nipples may become dry after surgery. You may use an ointment such as Aquaphor to help with this.

- You may experience a loss of sensation or increased sensitivity in the nipples following surgery. Usually, both of these improve with time. Rarely, numbness is permanent.

- You may have minimal watery drainage from the incisions during the first couple of days or weeks after surgery. This is more likely to occur at the points where two incisions meet, such as the junction of the vertical incision with the incision along the crease of the breast, or at the junction of the vertical incision with the incision around the areola. Placing gauze along these areas after surgery will keep them clean.

- You need to remember that the shape of the breasts immediately after surgery is not their final shape once completely healed. Initially, the breasts may appear slightly wide. Usually, they develop a more natural shape over the course of 6–12 months.

- During the first year or two of healing, you may feel areas of thickening along the scars, especially the scars along the breast crease. These will soften over time.

- You may feel areas of firmness within the breast tissue. These may simply be areas of scar or fat necrosis (hardening of the fatty tissue due to an inadequate blood supply). However, they must be examined by your surgeon, as the firm areas may represent an abnormal growth that requires further evaluation.

HOW DO I CARE FOR MYSELF AFTER BREAST REDUCTION SURGERY?

- Most surgeons use drains, one drain per breast. You will be taught how to manage the drains as you will go home with them. You will need to empty drains and record the amount of drainage. Based on the amount of drainage, the drains will be removed by your surgeon during the first 24–72 hours after surgery.

- Some surgeons do not recommend showering while the drains are in place, while other surgeons permit it. You may shower as soon as the drains are removed, or once your surgeon recommends that you do so. However, the breasts should not be soaked in a bathtub, swimming pool, or whirlpool for a minimum of four weeks, or until all of the wounds have completely closed.

- You will be wrapped in an Ace bandage or a surgical brassiere after surgery to help with breast compression. After approximately one week, patients find sports bras that zip in the front to be very comfortable. The sports bra must provide compression but not be excessively tight so as to minimize the potential for blistering. Your surgeon will advise you when you can wear a regular bra.

- The greatest discomfort will be within the first 24–48 hours after surgery. You should limit vigorous arm motion during that time. You should continue to avoid vigorous arm motion that requires excessive pushing, pulling, lifting, or over-the-head arm movements during the first two weeks after surgery.

- You may have surgical tape (Steri-strips) over the incisions. These strips are usually left in place for approximately two weeks. They further protect the incisions and will stay in place even with showering. Most surgeons prefer to let these fall off by themselves rather than actively remove them.

- Expect your breasts to be sore, swollen, and bruised. Over the course of the first week, the bruising may gravitate down toward the rib cage. The use of cold compresses during the first three days and warm compresses after that period of time may be helpful. You should not use ice or heat on the breast area without first checking the temperature of the compresses with your hand. The breasts will not have normal sensation after surgery, and you need to be careful not to burn your skin.

- Early on, if you experience increased sensitivity of the nipples, covering the area with an ointment such as Aquaphor and a non-adherent gauze will help.

- If you experience slight watery drainage from the incision sites, cover these with a non-adherent gauze to keep them clean.

- You need to monitor your breasts during the first week for any evidence of internal bleeding or infection. You need to notify your surgeon if you experience any of the following symptoms:

  o Signs of internal bleeding:

    1. Significantly asymmetrical swelling
    2. Excessive asymmetrical pain
    3. Bilateral pain not responding to pain medication
    4. Sudden increase in the degree of bruising
    5. Excessive firmness along a localized area of either breast

  o Signs of infection:

    1. Spreading redness along the breast
    2. A foul odor along the incisions

3. Pus from the incision site
4. Excessive warmth along the breast
5. Excessive localized tenderness along the breasts

- Although we know that we are not perfectly symmetrical in our appearance and accept some asymmetry as normal, we need to understand that our symptoms and signs of healing will also be slightly asymmetrical. There will always be a slight degree of asymmetry in the two breasts in terms of bruising, pain, and swelling. However, just as a great deal of asymmetry in our appearance is abnormal, a great degree of asymmetry in how we are recovering is abnormal. Generally speaking, you should experience a comparable degree of bruising, pain, and swelling in the two breasts. If you see significant differences between the two, you need to notify your surgeon.
- You may resume driving once you are no longer taking pain medication and you are comfortable moving your arms.
- It is very important that you take the prescribed antibiotic to help prevent infection.
- You should check with your surgeon before resuming any aerobic or weightlifting exercise program.

WHEN IS THE RIGHT TIME FOR A BREAST REDUCTION?

- Women present for breast reductions at many different points in life.
- They may present during or just after completing puberty if they experienced a significant growth in their breasts. Usually, these young women are very self-conscious of the size of their breasts and are often unable to wear youthful clothing or participate in a variety of sports. They generally complain of difficulty maintaining good posture and limited exercise tolerance, even though they may not yet have developed the back, shoulder, and neck pain due to the excess weight of the breasts. In these young patients, it is important to be certain that their breasts have completed growth prior to undergoing a breast reduction.
- Women may present much later in life when they have developed physical changes due to the weight of the breasts and can no longer tolerate excess weight. Usually, they present with neck and back pain, limited exercise tolerance, skin irritation under the breasts due to sagging, painful shoulder grooving due to

heaviness of the breasts on the bra straps, and difficulty performing adequate self–breast examinations for cancer detection due to breast size.

- Ideally, women would undergo a breast reduction when they begin to experience the side effects of the enlarged breasts and prior to developing advanced stages of these side effects.

19

Breast Lift (Mastopexy)

WHAT IS A BREAST LIFT?

- It is a surgical procedure to treat a condition called *mammary ptosis*, which means "falling breasts."
- Sagging results from loss of skin elasticity and/or loss of fullness in the breast tissue.
- These changes sometime follow pregnancy, breast-feeding, or weight loss, or occur as a natural course of aging.
- As the skin loses its elasticity, and the breasts lose volume, they begin to lose their shape; they sag, and the nipple begins to shift downward (Fig. 19.1).
- In a youthful breast, the nipple is found above the level of the breast crease.
- There are four degrees of ptosis that are described based on position of the nipple relative to the crease under the breast.

  - As the breast loses volume, it is first noted along the upper part of the breast without lowering of the nipple. This is called *pseudo-ptosis*, which literally means "false falling" since the nipple has not shifted.
  - With increasing sagging in the breasts, the nipple begins a downward descent.

    1. *Grade I ptosis* is when the nipple has dropped to the level of the breast crease.

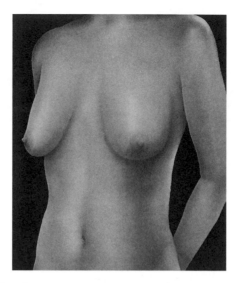

Figure 19.1.   As the skin loses its elasticity and the breasts lose volume, they begin to lose their shape, and the nipple begins to shift downward. (Courtesy American Society of Plastic Surgeons.)

    2. *Grade II ptosis* is when the nipple has dropped somewhat below the breast crease.

    3. *Grade III ptosis* is when the nipple has dropped to the lowest point of the breast.

WHAT DOES BREAST LIFT SURGERY ACCOMPLISH?

- It will raise the nipple and areola to a higher position.
- It will reshape the breasts for a more youthful contour, position, and appearance.
- If necessary, it will reduce the size of an enlarged areola (dark skin around the nipple).
- If the breasts are small or have lost volume after pregnancy or weight loss, breast implants may be inserted in conjunction with a breast lift in order to increase firmness and add fullness to the breasts.
- Although all sagging breasts may be lifted, patients with very large, heavy breasts may benefit from a small reduction as well as a breast lift.

WHERE ARE THE INCISIONS, AND ARE THERE SCARS ASSOCIATED WITH BREAST LIFT SURGERY?

- All breast surgery leaves scars.
- Different degrees of sagging require different types of lifting procedures and incisions, leaving the woman with either limited or extensive scars.
- Typically, the incisions and scars fall into one of four categories:
  - Along the upper segment of the areola (semi-circular incision)
  - Around the entire circular border of the areola (circular incision)
  - Around the entire circular border of the areola, extending from the areola down to the level of the breast crease ("lollipop" incision)
  - Around the entire circular border of the areola, extending from the areola down to the level of the breast crease, and along the level of the breast crease (anchor-shaped incision)

HOW IS A BREAST LIFT PERFORMED IN CASES OF PSEUDOPTOSIS?

- Since the nipple is in the youthful position and the issue is loss of breast volume, the treatment of choice for pseudoptosis is placement of a breast implant. This enhances the breast volume and shape with minimal scarring.
- There is usually no need to remove skin, and consequently, there are no additional incisions other than the one used for placement of the implant. (See Chapter 17 for a discussion of incisions and implant position placement.)

HOW IS A BREAST LIFT PERFORMED IN CASES OF GRADE I PTOSIS?

- Since the nipple is at the level of the breast crease and there is loss of breast volume, the two issues that must be addressed are raising the nipple and replacing volume.
- If the patient wants to maintain the same breast size or only minimally increase it, a very small implant may be used to enhance the volume and contour of the breast. The nipple is then raised simply by removing a crescent of the tissue above the areola (pink/brown area of skin around the nipple), thereby lifting it into the higher position. The scar is limited to the upper segment of the edge of the areola and is not easily visible. There are no

scars along the breast skin. The crescent lift should not be used to lift the nipple more than one or two centimeters. Otherwise, it will distort the areola.

DO PATIENTS WITH GRADE I PTOSIS HAVE ANY ALTERNATIVES TO AVOID A BREAST LIFT?

- Yes. If these patients wish to have an increase in the breast volume of at least one cup size, use of a slightly larger implant will usually achieve minor lifting by itself, without the need for tissue removal above the areola.

HOW IS A BREAST LIFT PERFORMED IN CASES OF GRADE II PTOSIS?

- Since the nipple has dropped below the breast crease and there is loss of volume, this degree of ptosis almost always requires removal of skin both above and below the nipple.
- If there is enough breast volume, and the patient desires a lift without breast enlargement, three possible incisions may be used.
  - A keyhole-shaped incision is made directly above the areola and carried down along the lower pole of the breast. The surgeon then works through that incision to remove the excess skin from the upper and lower parts of the breasts. The nipple and areola are repositioned to a higher, more youthful position (Fig. 19.2). As the vertical part of the skin incisions is closed, the breast mound is lifted to a higher position. The final scar surrounds the areola and extends vertically along the lower pole of the breast. This is the "lollipop" scar.
  - If there is much more skin to remove, the procedure described above is used, but there is an extension of the incision along the breast crease to remove additional skin (Fig. 19.3). This results in an anchor-like scar (Fig. 19.4). The final scar surrounds the areola, extends vertically along the lower pole of the breast and along the breast crease (Fig. 19.5). This is essentially the same as the incisions used for a breast reduction.
  - Another type of breast lift, known as a Benelli lift, may be used with more limited scarring. This places the entire scar within the limits of the areola. The excess skin above and below the nipple is removed through a donut-shaped skin excision surrounding the areola. Using a special non-dissolvable stitch, the larger circle of the donut is cinched in toward the smaller circle of the donut, which is the edge of the areola. The nipple is lifted, since more skin is removed from the upper part of the breast than from the lower part. Although this

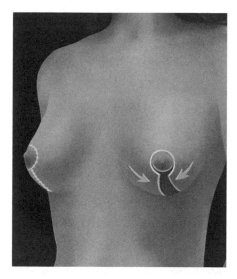

Figure 19.2. The nipple and areola are repositioned to a higher and more youthful position. (Courtesy American Society of Plastic Surgeons.)

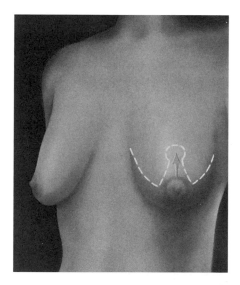

Figure 19.3. The incisions for a breast lift can vary, from those only along the upper areola, those encircling the areola and extending vertically along the midline of the breast, and those that also include an incision along the breast crease. (Courtesy American Society of Plastic Surgeons.)

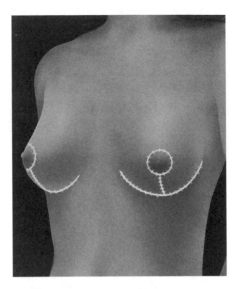

Figure 19.4. The most extensive breast lifts result in an anchor-like scar. (Courtesy American Society of Plastic Surgeons.)

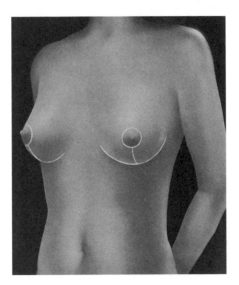

Figure 19.5. The final scar for these extensive breast lifts surrounds the areola and extends vertically along the lower pole of the breast and along the breast crease. (Courtesy American Society of Plastic Surgeons.)

may seem like a very attractive alternative to the keyhole incision, there are several limitations to the Benelli lift.

1. The stitch used to cinch in the breast tissue may break and lead to excessively enlarged and badly positioned areolas.

2. There is a "de-projection" of the nipple. Normally, the nipple is at the greatest point of projection alongthe surface of the breast. The Benelli lift flattens this natural projection. This is most noticeable on a profile view of the breasts. However, this de-projection may be desirable in patients whose areola projects too far from the surface of the breast.

3. There is not as much control over the shape of the breast as there is with the keyhole incision. Depending upon the patient's breast shape, the Benelli lift may lead to a boxy contour to the breast.

o In both the keyhole and Benelli breast lifts, patients may have a breast implant placed under the chest muscle to help improve the volume of smaller breasts.

DO PATIENTS WITH GRADE II PTOSIS HAVE ANY ALTERNATIVES TO AVOID THE SCARS ASSOCIATED WITH THESE LIFTING PROCEDURES?

- Often, patients with Grade II ptosis ask if placing an implant above the muscle will fill out the deflated tissue and correct the sagging without all of the scars associated with the lift. They need to be aware that this is not an ideal treatment. Although this typically adds volume and provides a minimal lift, it does not usually place the nipple back into its fully uplifted position, and the weight of the implant contributes to further breast sagging over time.

- Patients with Grade II ptosis who are unwilling to accept the scars associated with a breast lift should not rely on the implants to improve their condition. They should understand that placing an implant behind sagging breast tissue in order to fill it out will often simply create a larger sagging breast.

HOW IS A BREAST LIFT PERFORMED IN CASES OF GRADE III PTOSIS?

- In these cases, the nipple has dropped to the lowest part of the breast or is pointing downward from the breast, and there is usually a significant loss of breast volume. This degree of ptosis almost always requires considerable upward shifting of the nipple and an equally substantial removal of skin. This type of patient will almost always require the keyhole-shaped incision resulting in the anchor-like scar described above.

- The majority of these patients benefit from placement of a small breast implant behind the chest muscle to provide some upper pole fullness, as this is frequently missing in advanced stages of ptosis. Larger implants may be used to enhance the overall breast size if so desired by the patient.

IS BREAST LIFT SURGERY VERY PAINFUL?

- Generally, the greater the extent of surgery, the greater the discomfort.
- If breast implants are used in addition to the breast lift, patients will experience more pain than when the breast lift is performed alone.
- If the breast lift is performed without breast implants, patients report a mild, stinging-type pain along both breasts that diminishes over the subsequent two days following surgery.
- As would be expected, there is more discomfort if breast implants are used and placed behind the muscle.
- Much of the pain from a breast lift subsides after the first 48 hours following surgery.
- The pain should be easily controlled with the prescribed pain medication.

WHAT TYPE OF ANESTHESIA IS RECOMMENDED DURING BREAST LIFT SURGERY?

- The more limited breast lift, such as the crescent lift, may be performed under local anesthesia or under local anesthesia with sedation (twilight anesthesia).
- All other types of lifting procedures, especially those incorporating the use of breast implants, require more involved surgery. In these cases, general anesthesia is preferred by most surgeons.

WHEN ARE THE SUTURES REMOVED?

- Many surgeons use dissolvable sutures. These generally dissolve over the course of two weeks.
- If non-dissolvable sutures are used, these are removed within the first two weeks.

WHAT CAN I EXPECT AFTER BREAST LIFT SURGERY?

- When you awaken in the recovery room, you will have a dressing around the chest. This will consist of gauze and Ace wraps, or possibly a surgical brassiere.
- Usually, all of your incisions will be covered with surgical tape (Steri-strips) to further protect them. These strips fall off within the first two weeks after surgery. Most surgeons recommend that the patient not remove these tapes, as they are protecting the incisions and will fall off by themselves.
- You can expect to have bruising and swelling. The extent of both will vary proportionately with the extent of the lift. Generally, your bruising will be visibly worse at 48 hours after surgery than immediately after the procedure. In breast lift cases involving breast implants, the bruising is greater and may gravitate downward along the rib cage. The bruising and swelling will diminish over the subsequent weeks following surgery.
- During the first two weeks after surgery, you can expect:
  - Soreness along the entire breast area
  - Numbness along the breast skin
  - Numbness or increased sensitivity in the nipple area
  - Burning sensation in the nipple area
  - If the breasts feel numb, you may experience a tingling sensation or sharp twinges as the nerves are recuperating from surgery.
- Usually, all of these symptoms improve with time.
- The skin of the breasts and nipples may become dry after surgery. Liberal use of an ointment such as Aquaphor will alleviate this.
- With the more extensive breast lift procedures, there may be a minimal clear, yellow drainage from the incisions. This is more likely to occur at the points where two incisions meet, such as the junction of the vertical incision with the incision along the crease of the breast, or the junction of the vertical incision with the incision around the areola. This clear drainage usually stops during the first week or two after surgery.
- It is important to realize that the shape of the breasts immediately after breast lift surgery is not their final shape once they are completely healed.

- If implants are used with the breast lift and placed behind the muscle, it will take several months for them to drop into place, and initially, the breast mound will seem high.

- If implants are not used and you have undergone a Benelli- or anchor-type breast lift, the breasts may initially appear slightly wide or "boxy." They will take on a more natural shape over the course of 6–12 months.

- If a crescent-type breast lift is performed, the areola may initially appear slightly oblong. Although this improves with time, it may not completely correct itself if an attempt was made to lift the areola more than one or two centimeters.

- It is also important to realize that the scars will change significantly over time. All of the scars start out very thin and begin to get slightly thicker as healing progresses. If you underwent the anchor-type breast lift, the scar thickening is most noticeable along the scars within the breast crease. Although this thickening may last one to two years, it will soften over time. The incision around the areola and vertical incision along the front of the breast typically heal with a relatively finer scar. If you underwent the Benelli breast lift, you will experience a bunching of the skin at the junction of the skin and areola, since a larger circle is cinched toward the smaller circle. This usually improves over the course of months and may take as long as one year to significantly resolve.

HOW DO I CARE FOR MYSELF AFTER BREAST LIFT SURGERY?

- With your surgeon's consent, you may shower the day after surgery. However, the breasts should not be soaked in a bathtub, swimming pool, or whirlpool for a minimum of four weeks or if there is any persisting drainage from the incisions.

- If implants are used along with a breast lift, your greatest discomfort will be within the first 48–72 hours after surgery. If implants are not used, most of your discomfort will usually subside in the first 24 hours.

- Normally during the first few days after surgery, the breasts will be sore, swollen, and bruised. Over the course of the first week, bruising may gravitate down toward the rib cage. The use of cold compresses during the first three days and warm compresses after that period of time may be helpful. You should not use ice or heat on the breast area without first checking the temperature of the compresses with your hand. Your breasts will not have normal sensation after surgery, and you will need to be careful not to burn the skin.

- You need to monitor the breasts during the first week for any evidence of internal bleeding or infection. You need to notify your surgeon immediately if you experience any of the following symptoms:

  ○ Signs of internal bleeding, including:

    1. Significant difference in the extent of swelling between the two breasts
    2. Significant difference in the extent of pain between the two breasts
    3. Significant pain in both breasts not responding to pain medication
    4. Sudden increase in the degree of bruising
    5. Excessive firmness and tenderness along a localized area of one or both breasts

  ○ Signs of infection, including:

    1. Spreading redness along the breast
    2. A foul odor along the incisions
    3. Pus from the incision site
    4. Excessive warmth along the breast
    5. Excessive localized tenderness along the breasts

- You should limit your arm activity and avoid vigorous arm motion that requires intense pushing, pulling, lifting, or over-the-head arm movements during the first week.

- You will most likely have surgical tape (Steri-strips) over the incisions for approximately two weeks. The tape further protects the incisions and will stay on even with showering. Most surgeons prefer to let the tape fall off by itself rather than actively remove it.

- Initially after surgery, you may be wrapped in an Ace bandage or a surgical brassiere to help provide breast support and comfort. After approximately one week, you may find sports bras that zip in the front to be very comfortable. Your surgeon will advise you on an individual basis when a regular bra may be worn.

- If you experience increased sensitivity of the nipples, covering the area with an ointment such as Aquaphor and a non-adherent gauze will help.

- If you experience drainage from the incision sites, you may cover the areas with a non-adherent gauze to keep them clean.

- It is very important that you take the prescribed antibiotic to help prevent infection.

- You may resume driving once you are no longer taking pain medication.
- You should check with your surgeon before resuming any aerobic or weightlifting exercise program.

WHEN IS THE RIGHT TIME FOR A BREAST LIFT?

- Women usually present for a breast lift after childbearing, breast-feeding, significant weight loss, or simply changes due to aging.
- Young women finishing puberty may develop ptosis that warrants a breast lift without having experienced any of the above changes; however, this is less common.
- In these young patients, it is important to be certain that their breasts have completed growth prior to having them undergo a breast lift.

WHAT ARE THE LIMITATIONS OF BREAST LIFT SURGERY?

- This surgery cannot lift the breasts without scars. The greater the extent of ptosis, the greater the extent of the scars.
- Breast lifts cannot eliminate all stretch marks on the breast.
- All humans are asymmetrical, and symmetry should not be expected from these procedures.

IS THERE ANY EFFECT ON THE INCIDENCE OF BREAST CANCER IN PATIENTS WHO HAVE UNDERGONE A BREAST LIFT?

- The incidence of breast cancer is neither increased nor decreased.
- Physical examinations and mammograms are not usually affected, although some scar tissue will be present.
- A mammogram is usually recommended approximately 6–12 months after surgery to establish a new baseline for later reference.
- After surgery, you should continue undergoing mammograms according to the following schedule, unless otherwise dictated by your physician or family history:

  o Age 35-40: Screening mammogram
  o Over age 40: Mammogram once a year

WHO NEEDS A MAMMOGRAM PRIOR TO BREAST LIFT SURGERY?

- Women who are ages 35 to 40 and have never had a mammogram
- Women over the age of 40 and who have not had a mammogram within the year prior to the breast lift
- Women who have had an abnormal mammogram or a family history of breast disease
- Women who have abnormal findings on a breast examination

HOW LONG WILL THE EFFECT OF A BREAST LIFT LAST?

- Although the nipple has been repositioned and skin has been removed, subsequent breast sagging may occur as the result of aging, loss of skin elasticity, weight loss, pregnancy, menopause, and the effect of gravity on the remaining breast tissue.
- The rate at which future breast sagging occurs depends upon the patient's tissue quality, lifestyle, and the extent of the procedure performed. Generally, patients with thicker skin and dense breast tissue, who maintain a constant weight and consistently wear a brassiere, will experience a longer-lasting effect from the breast lift.
- Placement of an implant in front of the muscle will cause a faster degree of sagging due to the extra weight behind the breast tissue and the effects of gravity. This is somewhat better with placement of implants behind the chest muscle, but the weight of implants will always have some effect on the degree of sagging.

20

Correction of Inverted Nipples

WHAT IS AN INVERTED NIPPLE?

- A normal nipple projects outward from the apex of the breast. An inverted nipple describes the condition in which the nipple points inward, not outward. Generally, it is due to shortening of the milk ducts within the breast.
- It may occur in both men and women.
- It may affect one or both nipples.
- This condition is generally noted when the breasts develop, and continues throughout the individual's life.
- There is no health risk associated with having inverted nipples. *However*, if a normal nipple suddenly becomes inverted, it is important to establish that there is not an underlying cause within the breast tissue for this change. Certain tumors (benign or malignant) can develop under the nipple and may pull on the ducts, creating an inverted appearance. This condition needs to be evaluated by a qualified physician immediately.

WHAT DOES SURGERY ACCOMPLISH FOR INVERTED NIPPLES, AND HOW IS IT PERFORMED?

- It allows release of the nipple tissue so that it can project outward.
- Many different techniques are used, depending on the patient's needs.
- Generally, it involves making an incision within the nipple and areola (the brown area of skin around the nipple), dividing the ducts, and suturing the nipple tissue in an outward position.

ARE THERE ANY SCARS WITH CORRECTION OF INVERTED NIPPLES?

- As with all surgery, there are scars. These are limited to the area of the areola and nipple. As such, they are not typically very prominent.

IS THIS SURGERY VERY PAINFUL?

- Patients describe the pain as a mild-to-moderate stinging or burning pain. It is easily controlled with the prescribed pain medication.

WHAT TYPE OF ANESTHESIA IS RECOMMENDED FOR CORRECTION OF INVERTED NIPPLES?

- The incisions and necessary dissection are quite limited, and many patients tolerate this procedure under local anesthesia alone.
- If patients are apprehensive, twilight or general anesthesia may be used.

WHAT CAN I EXPECT AFTER SURGERY?

- Immediately after surgery, you will not have much sensation in the nipple due to the local anesthetic used. Over the first one to two hours, a mild to moderate pain develops along the nipple and surrounding tissues. This diminishes significantly during the first two to three days.
- On average, most people report 5–10 days of very mild soreness.
- During the first four to six weeks after surgery, the nipples may be overly sensitive or slightly numb.
- There will be swelling and bruising, but these are limited to the anterior portion of the breast and usually resolve over the course of one to two weeks.
- There is a possibility of permanent loss of sensation to the nipples.
- Since the ducts are cut in order to release the nipple tissue, the patient should not expect to be able to breast-feed after correction of the inverted nipple.

HOW DO I TAKE CARE OF MYSELF AFTER THIS TYPE OF SURGERY?

- During the healing phase, you need to protect the nipple in order to prevent it from becoming inverted again.

- You should avoid placing pressure against the nipple during the first four weeks after surgery. This is best achieved by using a thick gauze dressing with a cutout segment for the nipple inside the brassiere. In addition, you should avoid wearing tight brassieres that place a significant amount of pressure against the nipple.

- Most surgeons use dissolvable sutures, eliminating the need for suture removal. It is a good idea to keep the incision covered with a protective ointment such as Aquaphor until all sutures are dissolved.

- It is not uncommon for the nipple to become dry after this initial healing phase. You should continue applying an ointment such as Aquaphor or a gentle moisturizer such as Eucerin Body Lotion until the dryness resolves.

- The incisions within the nipple typically heal without a noticeable scar. Early on, you may experience a slight thickening of the scar. This is best treated with simple massage of the scar and surrounding skin for a few minutes each day.

21

Breast Reduction in Men (Gynecomastia Surgery)

Although gynecomastia affects men, it is important to discuss this condition in a book written for women. As women, men come into our lives as fathers, brothers, companions, husbands, and sons. Women should be aware of gynecomastia and should understand that it is very common and, if persistent, is readily treatable.

WHAT IS GYNECOMASTIA?

- Gynecomastia comes from the Greek term meaning "woman-like breasts" (Fig. 21.1). The term was introduced by Galen in the second century AD.
- It is very common and thought to affect 65 percent of boys in the 14-to-15-year age group and up to 30 percent of older men.
- Generally, it develops during early puberty and in many cases resolves after puberty. The incidence drops to less than 10 percent in boys over 17 years of age and begins to rise again after middle age.
- In the majority of time, gynecomastia occurs without a known cause and is a normal finding. However, it can be associated with an underlying disease at any age and warrants evaluation by a qualified physician.
  - Causes that must be ruled out include, but are not limited to:
    1. An increase in estrogen or a decrease in androgens
    2. Deficiency in androgen receptors
    3. Testosterone imbalance

   4. Pituitary gland tumors
   5. Adrenal gland tumors
   6. Prostate tumors
   7. Colon tumors
   8. Lung tumors
   9. Testicular disease
      Testicular tumors
      Testicular malfunction
  10. Thyroid disease
  11. Liver disease
      Hepatitis
      Cirrhosis
  12. Congenital syndromes
      Kleinfelter syndrome

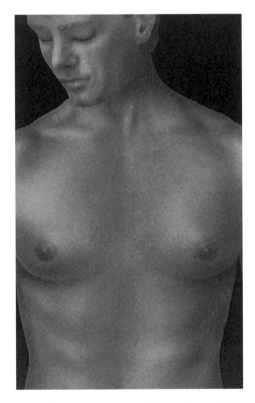

Figure 21.1. Many men have gynecomastia—enlarged, female-like breasts—caused by excess glandular tissue or fat. (Courtesy American Society of Plastic Surgeons.)

- Certain prescription and recreational drugs play a role in the development of gynecomastia.

  ○ Marijuana and heroin are known to potentially lead to gynecomastia.
  ○ The prescription drugs thought to contribute to gynecomastia include:

    1. Spirinolactone
    2. Tagamet
    3. Phenobarbital
    4. Antihypertensive drugs
    5. Steroids

ARE THERE DIFFERENT DEGREES OF GYNECOMASTIA?

- Many different classifications of gynecomastia have been developed. The most clinically useful classification defines the degree of gynecomastia according to the surgical approach needed.[1]

Grade I

- A localized button of breast tissue concentrated behind and around the areola without skin excess. The chest is not fatty, and the gynecomastia is very well-defined.

Grade II

- Diffusely enlarged breast tissue on a fatty chest with slight skin excess. The gynecomastia is not localized and does not have well-defined borders.

Grade III

- Diffuse gynecomastia on a fatty chest with moderate-to-severe excess skin.

HOW IS GYNECOMASTIA TREATED?

- If the gynecomastia is due to marijuana or prescription drugs, discontinuing these may help the condition.
- If gynecomastia develops during early puberty, it is best to allow the adolescent to complete puberty prior to any type of surgical intervention, as the condition may resolve on its own.
- If the gynecomastia persists after puberty and is not due to any type of drugs, then it is treated with surgery.

WHAT DOES GYNECOMASTIA SURGERY ACCOMPLISH?

- The procedure removes the fat and breast (glandular) tissue from the breast.
- In extreme cases, the skin may also need to be removed. This was quite common in the past. Since the introduction of ultrasonic liposuction for treatment of gynecomastia, the need for skin removal has decreased.
- Surgery results in flatter, firmer, and better-contoured breasts.

HOW IS SURGERY FOR GYNECOMASTIA PERFORMED?

- There are four possible approaches to the treatment of gynecomastia.

Ultrasonic Liposuction

- Since its introduction in the United States in the 1990s, ultrasonic liposuction has become a preferred approach to treatment of gynecomastia by many plastic surgeons.
- It allows removal of the excess fat and breast tissue through two very small incisions (3–4 mm each) placed within the circumference of the areola. The entire procedure is carried out through these incisions (Figs. 21.2, 21.3).
- The ultrasound energy helps the skin of the breast retract back, thereby significantly decreasing the potential need for skin removal (see Chapter 20).
- Adequate contouring of the fatty tissue located in the underarm area is also possible with this technique.

Direct Surgical Excision

- This technique allows the removal of the breast gland tissue and fatty tissue through an incision made within the lower one-third to one-half of the areola.
- Although this removes the extra tissue within the breast, it does not always provide adequate contouring of the excess tissue often found in the underarm area.
- If there is a significant amount of breast tissue that is directly removed, there may be excess skin that does not shrink back. This often necessitates direct excision of the skin through a separate incision.

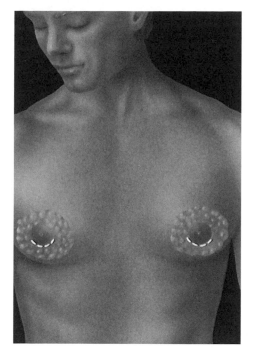

Figure 21.2. Glandular tissue must be cut out, usually through a small incision near the edge of the areola. (Courtesy American Society of Plastic Surgeons.)

- Most plastic surgeons prefer to consider skin excision as a secondary procedure only after adequate healing has occurred from the breast tissue excision. The breast skin may continue to improve up to one year after the initial procedure, and the need for direct skin excision may diminish over time, eliminating the need for a long scar.
- If the direct surgical excision technique is used, most surgeons will place a drain under the skin of the breast to collect any fluid that forms after surgery. This is usually removed within the first few days following surgery.

Direct Surgical Excision with Tumescent Liposuction

- Some surgeons will use a combination of direct surgical removal of the breast tissue and tumescent liposuction of the fatty tissue from the underarm region.

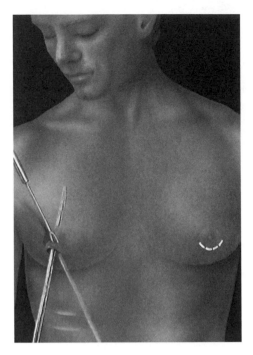

Figure 21.3. Fatty tissue can be removed by liposuction. A small, hollow tube is inserted through a tiny incision, leaving a nearly imperceptible scar. (Courtesy American Society of Plastic Surgeons.)

- This allows for improved contouring of the entire area, but it does not address the potential for excess skin along the breast.
- Tumescent liposuction is not as likely as ultrasonic liposuction to decrease the potential of redundant skin in cases of significant breast enlargement.
- As with direct excision alone, a drain may be placed to evacuate any excess fluid during the recovery period.

Breast Reduction with Removal of Breast Tissue and Simultaneous Removal of Skin

- This technique is reserved for cases of extreme gynecomastia.
- Unfortunately, it leaves extensive scars which are difficult to hide when undressed.
- Fortunately, this degree of gynecomastia is rare.

WHEN IS THE APPROPRIATE TIME FOR GYNECOMASTIA SURGERY?

- Gynecomastia is very common in pubertal boys and, in many cases, resolves on its own.
- If psychologically possible, most surgeons recommend treatment of gynecomastia after completion of puberty.

WHO IS A GOOD CANDIDATE FOR GYNECOMASTIA SURGERY?

- Boys who are in their late teens and have completed growth, and men of any age may be considered good candidates.
- Since much of the breast tissue consists of fat, the best candidates for surgery are those who are at or close to their ideal weight.

DOES THE PROCEDURE HURT?

- There is moderate pain involved, but most of the pain dissipates after the first 48 hours.
- After the first few days, patients will still experience tenderness and soreness in the breasts.
- During the healing process over the first several weeks, patients may feel excessive sensitivity of the nipples or numbness along the surgical site. This is normal and improves over time.
- There is a risk that the numbness of the nipples or breast skin may be permanent.

WHAT KIND OF ANESTHESIA IS RECOMMENDED FOR GYNECOMASTIA SURGERY?

- For very mild cases of gynecomastia treated with liposuction, local anesthesia alone may be used. For the majority of cases, twilight anesthesia or general anesthesia is recommended.

ARE THERE ANY SCARS?

- All of the described procedures leave scars.
- The scars from either the ultrasonic liposuction or the incision around the areola for direct excision of the breast tissue are minimal (Fig. 21.4).

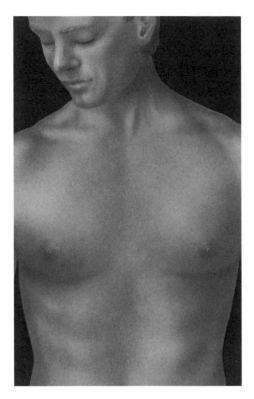

Figure 21.4. Following surgery for gynecomastia, the patient has a more masculine chest contour. (Courtesy American Society of Plastic Surgeons.)

- The only scars that are difficult to conceal are in patients requiring direct excision of skin.

WHAT CAN THE PATIENT EXPECT AFTER GYNECOMASTIA SURGERY?

- When patients awaken in the recovery room, they will have a compression-type dressing across their chest. Most surgeons use a zippered compression vest extending from the neck down to the mid-torso. This serves to control the swelling and prevents a seroma (blood/fluid collection under the skin) from forming. It also helps to support the skin and soft tissues firmly in place.
- If direct excision is used to remove breast tissue and/or skin, the patient will require a drain to be placed within each breast.

The drains remove the excess fluid that forms during healing after surgery. They are usually removed in the surgeon's office within 24–48 hours following the procedure. They may be left in place longer if their output suggests increased fluid production.

- If liposuction alone is used, usually there will not be any drains.
- Most of the pain is experienced in the first 24–48 hours.
- At 48 hours, the pain will decrease, but the swelling will reach its maximum.
- Most patients will remain bruised and swollen for approximately two weeks.
- The compression vest will help in controlling the swelling. It is recommended that patients wear the vest for two to four weeks, depending upon the type of procedure performed to treat the gynecomastia. In general, the more extensive the surgery, the longer the need for tissue support after surgery.
- Steri-strips (surgical tape) are usually placed on the incisions and are allowed to fall off by themselves.
- The initial surgical dressings are removed within the first 24–48 hours after surgery.
- Most surgeons use dissolvable sutures, but if non-dissolvable sutures are used, these are removed within the first week or two after surgery.
- The patient will notice a significant difference in the appearance of the breasts as soon as the surgical dressings are removed. However, he will not see the complete difference for 6–12 months due to minor swelling.

HOW DOES A PATIENT CARE FOR HIMSELF AFTER GYNECOMASTIA SURGERY?

- It is recommended that patients take approximately one week off from work.
- Excessive arm use during the first week is highly discouraged. Patients should minimize movements such as heavy pushing, pulling, and lifting for approximately four weeks.
- Avoiding sun exposure while bruised is critical, as it may lead to darkening of the bruised area; these pigment changes can last for many months or even years.

- Patients may have drains, which will help reduce bruising and the chance of a seroma (fluid collection under the skin). The timing of their removal depends upon how much fluid they are collecting. When the fluid level diminishes, the drains may be safely removed. They are usually removed within the first few days after surgery.

- If patients do not have drains or surgical padding that requires removal in their surgeon's office, they may remove the garment and shower the day after surgery. They may need some help when reapplying the garment the first few times. If patients have drains or additional padding that was applied during surgery, it is best to wait prior to showering until approved by their surgeon.

- When showering for the first time after surgery, some people become light-headed. It is best to take a short shower using warm water and consider having someone nearby just as a precaution.

- The compression garment should be worn at all times 24 hours a day for four weeks, except while showering. This is to help reduce the expected swelling and bruising that occurs after surgery.

- Driving may be resumed once patients are free of pain, feel comfortable, and are no longer using narcotic medications.

- Massaging is recommended to help contour and minimize any irregularities. Depending on the degree of the surgery and the patient's comfort, massaging is started after the first one to two weeks following surgery. Many massage specialists are experienced in lymphatic drainage massage and post-liposuction massage, and your surgeon's office may have some recommendations.

- Numbness and tingling in the surgical regions are normal sensations and may be expected to last up to 12–18 months. Feeling a sharp or tingling sensation after surgery is also expected and represents the nerves returning back to normal.

- Weight control is very important after surgery, as weight gain may lead to enlargement of the areas that underwent liposuction.

- Usually, any revision of the procedure should not be considered until 6–12 months after the surgery.

HOW LONG WILL THE EFFECTS OF GYNECOMASTIA SURGERY LAST?

- Although breast tissue and fat have been permanently removed, subsequent breast enlargement and sagging may occur as the result of weight gain, aging, loss of skin elasticity, future exposure to drugs (prescription or recreational), and the effects of gravity on the remaining breast tissue.

• Redevelopment and enlargement of breast tissue in men following breast reduction has been reported, but it is uncommon. If it does occur, it warrants an evaluation to rule out the medical causes discussed at the beginning of this chapter.

Aesthetic Body Surgery

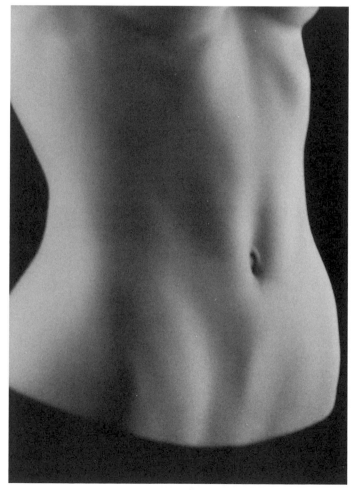

Stuart Rogers Photography

22

Liposuction

WHAT IS LIPOSUCTION?

- Liposuction is a technique to remove unwanted fat deposits from specific areas of the body (e.g., the neck, upper arms, abdomen, back, buttocks, hips, thighs, knees, calves and ankles; Figs. 22.1, 22.2).
- It allows the removal of fat using a small hollow metal tube (known as a cannula) under a controlled vacuum suction.
- Liposuction is not a method of weight reduction, but is a method of removing localized fat from areas that do not respond to dieting or exercise.
- Our size can be changed by weight reduction and exercise, but our shape stays relatively the same.
- Our shape is dictated by our bone structure, our muscle mass, and our fat deposits. The location and number of fat cells is determined by heredity (familial traits) and gender (male versus female).
  - We are born with a certain number of fat cells. The distribution of these fat cells throughout our body is determined by our genetics and gender. Some people inherit more fat cells in their hips and thighs relative to their abdomen. Others inherit more fat cells in their arms in comparison to their legs. In general, females inherit more fat cells in their hips and thighs ("saddle bags") while males inherit more fat cells in their abdomen and flanks ("love handles").
  - Growth and normal weight gain during childhood leads to an increase in the number of fat cells. However, the relative proportion of fat in different areas stays the same. So if an infant is born with more fat cells in the abdomen relative to the thighs, then as all of the fat cells in the body multiply and divide, there will be more fat

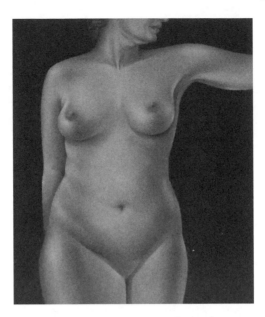

Figure 22.1. Women may have liposuction performed in many areas including: the neck, arms, abdomen, back, hips, thighs, and lower legs. (Courtesy American Society of Plastic Surgeons.)

cells in the abdomen than in the thighs. These fat cells multiply and divide, increasing in number until we complete puberty. After puberty, an increase in weight leads to an increase in the size of the fat cells. The exceptions to this are during pregnancy or extreme weight gain, in which the fat cells may begin to divide and multiply again.

o Since liposuction removes fat cells, the number of fat cells decreases, but the fat cells remaining may still increase in size if the individual gains weight.

WHAT DOES LIPOSUCTION ACCOMPLISH?

- It is designed to remove localized areas of fat and help contour one's shape.
- By removing the prominent areas of fat, it establishes more normal proportions between different areas of the body.
- Patients must continue to watch their diet and maintain adequate exercise after surgery.

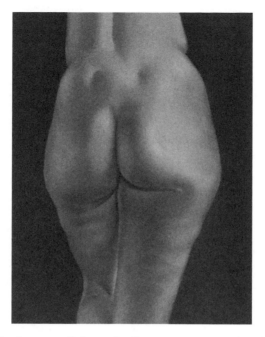

Figure 22.2.   The best candidates for liposuction are individuals who have normal weight with localized areas of excess fat—for example, in the buttocks, hips, and thighs. (Courtesy American Society of Plastic Surgeons.)

- If patients gain weight after liposuction, they will gain it more uniformly throughout the body, and it will not be as localized within their previous "problem areas."
- In general, patients will not see a huge weight difference on the scale, but will see a difference in inches. The average weight loss is approximately two pounds per liter of fat removed.

HOW IS LIPOSUCTION PERFORMED?

There are two types of liposuction that are routinely performed:

- Tumescent Liposuction
- Ultrasonic Liposuction

Although there is newer technology incorporating lasers in liposuction procedures, this is not widely practiced, and the potential applications, risks, and benefits are still being investigated. As such, we will limit our discussion to tumescent and ultrasonic liposuction.

How Is Tumescent Liposuction Performed?

- A small incision (3–4 millimeters) is made in the area adjacent to the localized fat pocket. The incision is just large enough to allow the cannula (a hollow instrument that pulls out the fat) into the tissues.
- At first, a tumescent solution that consists of saline (salt water) with medications (Lidocaine and Epinephrine) is injected into the fatty tissues of the area to undergo liposuction. The salt water distends the fatty layer. The medications allow the area to become numb and decrease the extent of bleeding.
- Once all areas are treated with this fluid, liposuction is performed.
- Liposuction is performed by using a hollow metal surgical instrument, known as a cannula, that is inserted through small skin incision(s) and is passed back and forth through the fatty tissues in the area being treated. The cannula is attached to a vacuum source, which provides the suction needed to remove the fat (Fig. 22.3).

How Is Ultrasonic Liposuction (also called Ultrasound Assisted Liposuction) Performed?

- This procedure is the same as the tumescent liposuction, with the addition of ultrasound energy to help in the breakdown of fat.
- After the tumescent solution is added to the fatty areas, an ultrasound probe (a thin metal probe able to transmit ultrasound energy at its tip) is inserted into the fatty areas and moved back and forth. Each area is treated for a period of multiple minutes with the ultrasound energy to help break down the fat.
- The level of ultrasound energy used and the length of time the ultrasound energy is applied to the tissue depend upon the specific area being treated, the amount of fat to be removed and the type of fat to be removed. Areas in which the fat is very dense fat (such as the back) require higher levels of ultrasound energy delivered for a longer period of time than areas in which the fat is less dense (such as the inner thighs). Areas containing a thicker fatty layer will require treatment with ultrasound energy for a longer period of time than thinner areas.
- Following treatment of the fatty areas with tumescent fluid and ultrasound energy, liposuction is performed as described above.

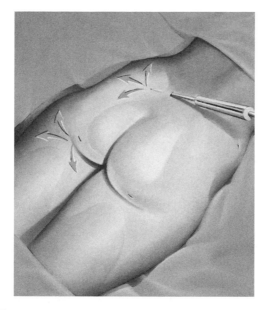

Figure 22.3. The surgeon inserts a cannula through small incisions in the skin. At the other end of the tube is a vacuum-pressure unit that suctions the fat. (Courtesy American Society of Plastic Surgeons.)

Are There Any Advantages to the Addition of Ultrasound Energy to Liposuction?

Ultrasound liposuction has several advantages over tumescent liposuction.

- It allows the removal of larger amounts of fat with less bleeding.
- It tackles areas of dense fat that were very difficult and unsuccessful to treat previously, such as the back.
- It allows more successful treatment of areas that previously underwent liposuction in which a revision is required. The dense scar tissue in these areas may make it difficult to perform additional liposuction using the tumescent technique alone. However, the use of ultrasound energy helps break down some of the scar tissue, allowing the liposuction cannula to then pass through the fat more easily.
- It improves the ability of the skin to shrink back following fat removal.

Are There Any Disadvantages to the Addition of Ultrasound Energy to Liposuction?

• Ultrasound liposuction should be performed only by surgeons who are well trained in this technique as it carries a risk of burning the skin.

• There have been cases reported of permanent change in the sensation of the skin following the use of ultrasound energy. Although this may occur with any type of surgical procedure and is not dangerous, patients should be aware that it is possible.

WHO ARE GOOD CANDIDATES FOR LIPOSUCTION?

• The best candidates for liposuction are individuals of relatively normal weight who have excess fat in certain body areas. These well-localized fat pockets are usually areas that have been resistant to diet and exercise.

• Having firm, elastic skin will result in a better final contour following liposuction. Excess or loose skin is less likely to re-drape smoothly over the treated area. If the skin does not re-drape sufficiently, it may require surgical removal as a secondary procedure.

WHAT ARE THE LIMITATIONS OF LIPOSUCTION?

• Liposuction cannot provide skin elasticity.

• The ability of the skin to shrink over the new contour is not completely predictable.

• Usually, younger patients have better skin elasticity than older patients, and the use of ultrasonic energy helps with skin retraction. However, the more fat that is removed from an area, the greater the difficulty for the skin to shrink back smoothly, regardless of patient age and use of ultrasound energy. This often results in surface irregularities following liposuction.

• All humans are asymmetrical, and symmetry may not result from liposuction.

• Liposuction alters one's shape but is not an answer to weight problems. Weight can be controlled only with diet and exercise.

• In general, liposuction itself will not improve areas of dimpled skin known as "cellulite."

- Body contour irregularities due to structures other than fat, such as muscle, muscle weakness, bone, cartilage, and intra-abdominal contents, cannot be improved by liposuction alone.

ARE THERE ANY SCARS?

- All surgery leaves scars. The external scars with liposuction are limited to the small incisions used for the passage of the cannulas.
- There will be internal scarring within the fat layer due to liposuction. This typically softens over time. If the scarring is excessive, it often will present as irregularities, depressions, or dimpling in the skin.

WHERE ARE THE INCISIONS PLACED?

- Typically, two incisions are necessary for each area to undergo liposuction. This allows passage of the cannulas in crisscross directions to allow a smoother removal of fat and minimize the potential for irregularities in the skin.
- Depending on the area to undergo liposuction, the incisions are placed within folds of skin whenever possible, or easily hidden, such as within the navel or within existing scars.

ARE THERE STITCHES?

- Most surgeons close the liposuction incisions using a single suture (stitch) per incision. These sutures may or may not be dissolvable. If not dissolvable, they are usually removed within the first week following surgery.

WHAT IS THE RECOVERY TIME?

- The recovery time depends on the area and degree of liposuction performed.
- It can vary from one day for limited liposuction (neck liposuction) to one week for more extensive liposuction (liposuction of the abdomen and hips or other combination areas).

DOES LIPOSUCTION HURT?

- Generally, the degree of pain depends on the extent of liposuction.
- There is usually an initial burning sensation that improves over the course of the first 24–48 hours. Following this period, the pain is best described as soreness and stiffness rather than significant discomfort.
- By the fifth day after liposuction, patients begin to feel far more comfortable and begin resuming many of their daily activities.

WHAT KIND OF ANESTHESIA IS RECOMMENDED DURING LIPOSUCTION?

- For limited areas of liposuction, local anesthesia may be used.
- For larger areas of liposuction or ultrasonic liposuction, either twilight or general anesthesia is recommended.
- Some physicians will use local anesthesia for larger areas of liposuction. However, this requires staging the procedure, as there is a limit to the amount of local anesthetic that may be used safely. If the patient is under general or twilight anesthesia, less local anesthetic is required.

WHAT CAN I EXPECT AFTER LIPOSUCTION?

- When you awaken in the recovery room, you will have a compression garment covering all of the areas that underwent liposuction (Fig. 22.4). Expect to feel a slight burning sensation over these areas as well as tightness from the garment.
- Many plastic surgeons use a product called "Topifoam" under the compression garment during the first few days after surgery. Topifoam consists of sheets of foam with a silicone layer that adheres to the skin. It provides additional compression and is thought to lead to lesser degrees of swelling and bruising.
- The compression garment is usually worn for 24 hours a day for a period of four to six weeks. It may be taken off to shower and to be washed.
- For the first 24 hours after surgery, you may notice some leaking of the saline solution tinged with blood from the small incisions. This may occur even if your incisions are closed with a suture.

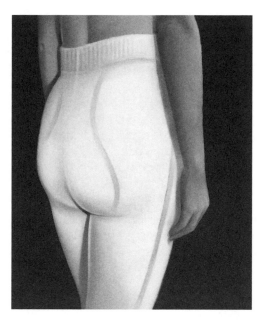

Figure 22.4. A compression garment covering the areas that underwent lipo-suction helps reduce swelling. (Courtesy American Society of Plastic Surgeons.)

- You should expect bruising and swelling to occur. Most of the bruising resolves over the first two weeks.
- The compression garment helps to control the extent of swelling.
- As you begin to ambulate and resume regular daily activities, the bruising and swelling gravitate downward (the effect of gravity). For example, following liposuction of the abdomen, the bruising and swelling gravitate to the pubic area; following liposuction of the thighs, the bruising and swelling gravitate to the knees and, sometimes, even to the ankles.
- In terms of recovery, every patient is different. On average, it takes most patients approximately one week to resume most of their daily activities following liposuction of one or two areas of the trunk. If multiple areas of the body undergo liposuction, a slightly longer recovery is likely.
- During the healing process, you may feel a burning sensation along the areas that underwent liposuction. You should also expect to feel twinges of pain, numbness, and tingling in those areas. This is normal, as the nerves are healing from surgery.

- You will find that your weight has increased during the first week after liposuction. This is due to the extra fluid given during the procedure and to the normal swelling after surgery. Patients who weigh themselves immediately after liposuction are sure to be disappointed.
- You will see a difference in the area that underwent liposuction as soon as your garment is removed for the first time after surgery. However, the immediate result is not the final result. Over the subsequent three to four weeks, you will notice a gradual but significant change in your contour. On average, it will take three months before you will see most of the result, and up to six months or one year before you see the complete result.
- Sometimes, patients experience episodes of slight disappointment or depression after surgery while waiting for the results. This will subside as you begin to look better and feel better.

HOW DO I CARE FOR MYSELF AFTER LIPOSUCTION?

- You should wear the compression garment 24 hours a day for four to six weeks, except while showering. This is to help reduce the expected swelling and bruising that occur after surgery.
- You may have some leaking of blood-tinged fluid from the liposuction incisions during the first 24–48 hours. During this period, it is recommended that you place towels or sheets underneath you when sleeping or sitting to protect your mattresses and furniture.
- If you have had extensive liposuction of the abdomen, you may have drains. These will help reduce bruising and the chance of a seroma (fluid collection under the skin). The drains will be taken out within several days after surgery. You will be taught how to take care of the drains while you have them. On a daily basis, you will need to record how much fluid the drains collect over the course of day. This will allow your surgeon to determine when the drains are ready to be removed.
- Your surgeon will give you specific instructions as to showering. In general, if you do not have drains or special padding, you may remove your garment and shower three to five days after surgery. You may need some help when reapplying the garment for the first few times. Do not remove the garment or foam if you have drains unless so instructed by your surgeon. Usually, your surgeon will remove the garment and foam when you are seen in

the office for the drain removal and instruct you on the timing of your first shower.

- When showering for the first few times after surgery, do not take lengthy showers or use very hot water. Since you will take your compression garment off to shower, you may feel light-headed due to a drop in your blood pressure. It is important to have someone nearby when showering for the first few times after you have undergone liposuction.

- Do not drive until you are free of pain and feel comfortable without narcotic medications.

- Avoid any strenuous activities (jogging, aerobics, tennis, golf, etc.) for two weeks. However, you must start walking the day after surgery, unless you have had liposuction of the calves or ankles.

- If you have had liposuction of your calves or ankles, you need to keep your legs elevated as much as possible when you are not ambulating. These areas are very prone to prolonged swelling, and elevating your legs during the first three or four weeks after surgery will be very helpful. Some plastic surgeons even recommend the use of compression machines designed to decrease swelling in the lower legs. These consist of boot-like devices that gently massage the lower legs using pulses of pressure. They are used by the patient when sleeping at night during the first month after surgery. These machines may be rented through a medical supply company.

- Massaging may be beneficial to help resolve the swelling and decrease the potential for prolonged firmness along the areas treated with liposuction. Usually, massaging is started once you can tolerate the pressure. This is within the first two weeks after surgery. Most plastic surgery offices refer their patients to massage professionals with experience in post-liposuction massage.

- Sometimes, you will require a revision of the area that underwent liposuction. Revisions should not be considered until 6–12 months after the surgery, as many of the visible surface irregularities are due to swelling and resolve on their own.

- Liposuction is a lifelong commitment. It is very critical to control your weight after surgery. Do not have the procedure if you know you cannot manage your weight. Patients who gain weight after liposuction are sure to be disappointed. Ideally, you would permit yourself a fluctuation of two to three pounds. You need to weigh yourself at least twice per week to be certain that you are not gaining weight. If you see that your weight is climbing, begin to increase your exercise and decrease your food intake. It is much easier to lose two pounds than it is to lose 20 pounds. Although this is simple common sense, many liposuction patients experience weight gain after liposuction because their "intrinsic scale" has been removed. For example, if a woman has disproportionately heavy thighs, then throughout her life, she knows if she has gained or lost weight based on the appearance of her thighs and how her clothes fit over her thighs. She is not usually looking at her abdomen or her arms to see what has happened to her weight. She has been conditioned to examine her thighs to judge her weight. Suddenly after surgery, her thighs are much thinner, and her clothes fit well. If she is not careful, she will not notice a slight weight gain because she is still monitoring her thighs. She has not been carefully looking at other parts of her body. Months later, when she weighs herself and sees that she gained 10 pounds, she notices that other areas are slightly larger.

WHEN IS THE RIGHT TIME FOR LIPOSUCTION?

- Liposuction should not be considered until the individual is an adult and has completed growth.
- It should not be considered as a method of weight loss or weight control.
- It is a good procedure for men and women who have areas of their body that have been unresponsive to diet and exercise.
- At the time of surgery, patients should be at a *stable* and reasonable weight. They should not be experiencing major fluctuations in their weight.
- Female patients considering liposuction of the abdomen should do so either prior to having any children or following the birth of their last child. The abdomen will undergo many changes during childbearing, and the full effect of liposuction may not be appreciated in the midst of this period.

HOW LONG WILL THE EFFECT OF LIPOSUCTION LAST?

- Reducing the populations of fat cells in an area will produce a contour alteration that is expected to be permanent. However, the size of the fat cells that are left behind is controlled by diet and exercise.

- If you gain weight, all of the fat cells in the body will increase in size and make the areas fuller.
- In order for the effect of liposuction to last, you must control your weight.
- Additional alterations in your body contour may occur as a result of aging, pregnancy, menopause, hormone imbalance, and a variety of other conditions. The only condition over which you can exert control is your weight.

23

Tummy Tuck (Abdominoplasty)

WHAT IS AN ABDOMINOPLASTY?

- This procedure involves the removal of excess skin and fat from the middle and lower abdomen. It also tightens the muscles of the abdominal wall that may have lost their tone due to pregnancy or significant weight fluctuations.
- Abdominoplasty is not a surgical treatment for being overweight.
- Patients who are overweight and who intend to lose weight should postpone all forms of body-contouring surgery until they have reached their goal weight and have been able to maintain their new weight for at least six months.
- Abdominoplasty procedures may be classified into two general types:
  - *Full Abdominoplasty*: This procedure addresses the extra skin, fat, and muscle both above and below the navel.
  - *Mini-abdominoplasty*: This procedure addresses the extra skin, fat, and muscle below the navel. The navel and tissue above the navel are not treated.

WHAT DOES AN ABDOMINOPLASTY ACCOMPLISH?

- It treats the abdominal bulge, creating a flat abdominal contour.
- It removes the excess skin and lower abdominal stretch marks that may have resulted from increased skin laxity following pregnancy or significant weight loss.
- It improves the resting tone of the abdominal muscles.

- It may be used to repair hernias that occur along the navel, and the abdominal muscle separation that occurs following pregnancy.

WHAT ARE THE LIMITATIONS OF AN ABDOMINOPLASTY?

- An abdominoplasty cannot completely eliminate stretch marks. A full abdominoplasty will remove the majority of the stretch marks below the navel, but not those above the navel. The appearance of the stretch marks above the navel improves because of the overall tightening of the tissues. Furthermore, many of these stretch marks are pulled lower along the abdomen, often to a position below the navel.
- Generalized obesity cannot be corrected. An abdominoplasty should never be used as a weight loss method in these conditions.
- An abdominoplasty does not change the fat along the flanks. This region is best served with liposuction. Depending on the amount of liposuction necessary, it may be performed either simultaneously with the abdominoplasty, or as a secondary procedure.
- Although it improves the resting abdominal muscle tone, an abdominoplasty will not increase the abdominal muscle strength.

HOW IS A FULL ABDOMINOPLASTY PERFORMED?

- A curved horizontal incision is made, extending from one hip bone down toward the pubic hair line up toward the opposite hip bone (Fig. 23.1).
- A second incision is made around the navel in order to leave it attached to its stalk (Fig. 23.2).
- The skin and fatty tissues are then elevated off the underlying abdominal muscles from the level of the pubic area all the way up to the lower part of the breastbone (Fig. 23.3).
- Once these tissues are elevated, a permanent suture (stitch) is used to tighten the muscles along the midline from the level of the breastbone all the way down to the pubic bone (Fig. 23.3).
- After tightening the muscles, the excess skin and fat are cut away, and a new opening is made for the navel (Fig. 23.4). The navel is then sewn in place.

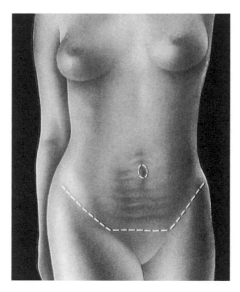

Figure 23.1. An incision just above the pubic area is used to remove excess skin and fat from the middle and lower abdomen. (Courtesy American Society of Plastic Surgeons.)

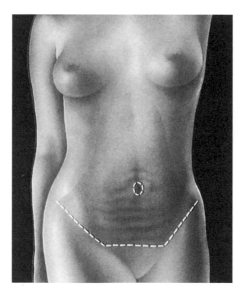

Figure 23.2. Skin is separated from the abdominal wall all the way up to the ribcage. (Courtesy American Society of Plastic Surgeons.)

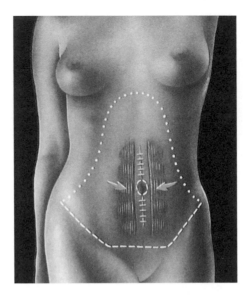

Figure 23.3. The surgeon draws underlying abdominal muscles together and stitches them, thereby narrowing the waistline and strengthening the abdominal wall. (Courtesy American Society of Plastic Surgeons.)

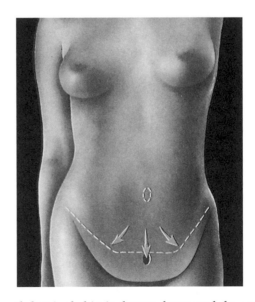

Figure 23.4. The abdominal skin is drawn down and the excess is removed. With a full abdominoplasty, a new opening is cut out for the navel. Both incisions are stitched closed. (Courtesy American Society of Plastic Surgeons.)

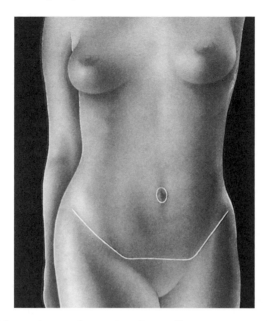

Figure 23.5. After surgery, the patient has a flatter, trimmer abdomen. Scars are permanent, but will improve with time. (Courtesy American Society of Plastic Surgeons.)

- The lower abdominal incision is then sewn closed (Fig. 23.5). Usually, several layers of tissue are sewn together to protect the repair and decrease the tension on the skin.
- Most plastic surgeons cover the abdominoplasty incision with surgical tape to further protect it during the healing period.
- Normally, the body forms fluid in the space that was created between the abdominal muscles and the elevated tissues. Drains are used under the tissue that was elevated to remove this fluid until the tissues re-adhere to the underlying muscles. Once the tissues re-adhere, the body stops forming the fluid. These drains are brought out through small openings in the pubic hair-bearing area. The drains are removed by the surgeon once the fluid diminishes. Usually, the drains are in place for several days. In some cases, the drain output may remain significant for a longer period of time, requiring the drains to be kept in place for more than one week.

HOW IS A MINI-ABDOMINOPLASTY PERFORMED?

- A horizontal incision is made just above the pubic hairline. The length of the incision depends on the extent of excess skin to be removed; the greater the amount of skin to be removed, the longer the incision.
- The skin and fatty tissues are then elevated from the underlying abdominal muscles up to the level of the navel.
- If needed, the muscles are then tightened along the midline from the level of the navel to the level of the pubic bone.
- The excess skin and fat are then cut away.
- The incision is closed with sutures in several layers of tissue, just as with a full abdominoplasty.
- The incision is usually covered with surgical tape for added protection during the healing period.
- Just as with a full abdominoplasty, drains are used to remove any fluid that forms in the space between the muscle and elevated tissues. Usually, the drains used with a mini-abdominoplasty are needed for a shorter period of time than those with a full abdominoplasty.

WHAT IS THE RECOVERY TIME?

- Everyone is different in terms of pain tolerance. Usually, most patients require two weeks of recovery following a full abdominoplasty and one week following a mini-abdominoplasty. Although you may be able to resume most activities of daily living after this initial period of time, you will not feel completely back to normal for several weeks.
- The critical factor in the length of recovery is the extent of muscle work performed during the abdominoplasty. If the muscles are not tightened, recovery is significantly shortened.

DOES AN ABDOMINOPLASTY HURT?

- You will have some pain. There are two types of pain following an abdominoplasty. There is pain along the incision, and there is pain due to the tightening of the abdominal muscles.

- The muscle pain may manifest as spasms or as tightness. The pain along the incision is usually described as a sharp or burning sensation. The muscle pain is the more intense of the two.

- As such, there is more pain associated with a full abdominoplasty than with a mini-abdominoplasty. In a full abdominoplasty, the muscle is tightened from the breastbone all the way down to the pubic bone. In a mini-abdominoplasty, the muscle is tightened from the level of the navel to the pubic bone.

- The most intense pain and muscle spasms occur during the first three to five days following surgery.

- Expect to be uncomfortable during these three to five days, but the pain medication and muscle relaxants prescribed by your surgeon should be sufficient to control the pain. If the pain is more than can be managed by the prescribed medications, you need to notify your surgeon.

WHERE ARE THE SCARS FOLLOWING AN ABDOMINOPLASTY?

- For a full abdominoplasty, there are two scars: the curved horizontal scar along the lower abdomen extending from hip bone to hip bone, and the scar around the navel.

- For a mini-abdominoplasty, there is only the curved horizontal scar along the lower abdomen.

- For both types of procedures, the length of the curved horizontal scar depends on the amount of excess skin and soft tissue to be removed.

WHAT KIND OF ANESTHESIA IS RECOMMENDED DURING AN ABDOMINOPLASTY?

- Most surgeons will recommend general anesthesia for either a full abdominoplasty or a mini-abdominoplasty.

- Twilight anesthesia (local anesthesia with sedation) may be used in a select number of cases, depending on the extent of surgery needed and the individual patient's degree of comfort.

- Some surgeons will recommend epidural or spinal anesthesia (similar to the type of anesthesia used during childbirth).

WHAT CAN I EXPECT AFTER AN ABDOMINOPLASTY?

- When you awaken in the recovery room, you will be in a semi-sitting position, with the head of the bed elevated and the knees bent. Most likely, you will have a binder wrapped around your abdomen for added support.

- Expect to feel tightness along the entire abdominal region when you awaken from surgery. This is from the muscle repair and removing the excess skin and fat. Also, you will experience a slight burning sensation along the incision.

- During the first two weeks after a full abdominoplasty, you may be more comfortable sleeping in a semi-sitting position with two to three pillows behind your head and one pillow under your knees. This decreases the amount of tension along your incision, which helps with the healing process. Since there is less tension along the incision with a mini-abdominoplasty, you may sleep in a more reclining position following these procedures.

- For the first few days after surgery, you will have drains to collect any excess fluid or serum that forms under the elevated abdominal tissue. You will be taught how to care for the drains and how to measure the fluid that they collect. Once the drain output diminishes to a safe level, the drains will be removed in your doctor's office.

- Most patients do not have significant bruising following an abdominoplasty, since the drains remove the blood-tinged fluid. If liposuction of other areas is performed at the same time, you should expect some bruising in those areas.

- You will have swelling after an abdominoplasty. This will occur along the abdomen and the pubic area. Although much of the swelling resolves after three months, there is residual swelling for up to one year.

- Once the drains are removed, many plastic surgeons switch the abdominal binder to a different compression garment that may be more comfortable and inconspicuous under clothing. The use of a compression garment helps control some of the swelling that occurs as a result of surgery.

- As you begin to ambulate after a full abdominoplasty, you may feel more comfortable walking slightly bent forward at the waist. This position decreases the tension along the abdominoplasty incision that may be experienced during the first two weeks following a full abdominoplasty. This tension is not usually experienced to an appreciable extent with a mini-abdominoplasty.

- During the healing process, you will feel a burning sensation along the incision line and twinges of pain along the upper and lower abdomen.
- You will have numbness along the upper and lower abdomen following a full abdominoplasty and along the lower abdomen following a mini-abdominoplasty. This numbness improves over time. You should expect to feel slight tingling along the abdomen as the nerves are healing from surgery. Sensation returns to most of the abdomen, but it will not be completely normal. Usually, patients will have permanent numbness along the incision.
- You will find that your weight has increased during the first few days following an abdominoplasty. This is due to the intravenous fluid given during the procedure and to the normal swelling after surgery. After the initial 24–48 hours following surgery, you will begin to void much of this extra fluid. As this occurs, your weight will decrease. Once the swelling begins to diminish, your weight should drop below your pre-surgical weight since some of your tissue was removed during the procedure.
- Although you will see an improvement in the contour of your abdomen immediately after surgery, you will appreciate a greater difference over the subsequent weeks to months. On average, it will take three months before you will see much of the results, and up to one year before you see the complete result.

HOW DO I CARE FOR MYSELF AFTER AN ABDOMINOPLASTY?

- You will have drains after surgery. The drains must be emptied with the drainage amount recorded daily, since this will determine the appropriate time for drain removal.
- You will be placed in a compression garment after surgery. This should be worn at all times except when showering for a minimum of four to six weeks.
- Usually, the incision will be covered with surgical tape (Steri-strips). The tape should be left in place until either it falls off by itself, or it is removed in your surgeon's office.
- Starting the day after surgery, you should walk at home as much as you can comfortably tolerate.
- You may begin activities of daily living, such as brushing your teeth, washing your face, and getting dressed, immediately after your surgery. Some surgeons allow their patients to shower while

they still have their drains, whereas others insist that the drains be removed prior to taking the first shower. It is best to check with your physician for guidelines with respect to showering.

- You may feel weak during the first two to three days following surgery. Eating a healthy diet is necessary to keep up your strength. It is also important to drink plenty of liquids (water, juice, Gatorade, etc.).

- During the first week, you may need assistance at home with getting up and down as well as changing your dressings or emptying your drains.

- Due to pain medication and inability to use your abdominal muscles, you will become constipated. It is best to take a proactive approach to counteract this. Non-prescription stool softeners (Dulcolax) or suppositories (Fleet's Glycerin Suppositories) may be used if you do not have a bowel movement in the first two days after surgery.

- When lying in bed for the first two weeks, use two pillows behind your back and one pillow under your knees. This keeps your back elevated and your knees bent, thereby decreasing the tension along the incision during the initial healing period. Some patients prefer to sleep in a recliner throughout this stage.

- Similarly, when walking during the first one to two weeks following surgery, it is beneficial to walk slightly bent forward at the waist so as to decrease the tension along the incision.

- You should avoid baths, whirlpools, and swimming pools during the first four weeks after an abdominoplasty, for two reasons. First of all, shower water is considered clean, while sitting water (baths, whirlpools, or swimming pools) is not. If you have an area along your incision or drain site that has not fully healed, sitting water is a setup for an infection. Secondly, sitting in a warm body of water for any length of time will contribute to swelling and is discouraged during the early healing period.

- You may resume light household duties and driving approximately two weeks after a full abdominoplasty, and approximately one week after a mini-abdominoplasty.

- You should not drive until you are off all prescription pain medication and muscle relaxants.

- It will take approximately two weeks after a full abdominoplasty and one week after a mini-abdominoplasty before you are feeling like yourself again. During this time, you should expect discomfort along the abdominal incision and along the muscle tightening. The prescribed pain medications and muscle relaxants should help with the discomfort.

- It will take approximately three to four weeks until you feel like you are moving freely and your clothes are fitting comfortably.

- Do not smoke after this procedure, as it will compromise circulation to the surgical site, causing severe complications. Smokers should stop smoking at least one month prior to and one month after surgery. If you are a smoker, you need to discuss this with your surgeon prior to surgery. Based on the extent of your smoking, your surgeon will determine how long you need to stop smoking before and after your abdominoplasty.

- If there is an incision around the navel, you need to clean it once daily with medicated soap and water and cover it with an ointment such as Aquaphor.

- Since you will not have normal sensation along the abdomen immediately after surgery, you should not use hot-water bottles or heating pads, as you may burn the skin.

- You should refrain from tanning and tanning beds for at least six weeks. The actual incisions should not be tanned until they are completely healed and faded. This is usually after the first one or two years. If a scar is exposed to the sun or to a tanning bed while it is still red or pink, it will become darker and potentially remain discolored long term.

- You may resume sexual intercourse four weeks after surgery if it is comfortable to do so.

- As a general guideline, you should avoid lifting anything heavier than five pounds during the first two weeks after surgery, ten pounds during the first six weeks after surgery, and 20 pounds during the first six months after surgery. Excessive lifting may strain and compromise the muscle repair.

- You should not strain the abdominal muscle repair for at least six months following an abdominoplasty. Although you are encouraged to walk immediately after surgery, you should not jog, swim, bicycle, lift weights, or participate in aerobic-type exercises such as tennis until given clearance by your surgeon. Under most circumstances, patients can gradually resume exercising six weeks after an abdominoplasty. However, specific abdominal exercises, such as sit-ups or abdominal crunches, should be avoided for approximately six months following surgery to prevent disruption of the muscle repair.

- It is very important that you take the prescribed antibiotic to help prevent infection.

HOW LONG WILL THE EFFECT OF AN ABDOMINOPLASTY LAST?

- The effect of the abdominoplasty should be permanent, since the excess skin and fat are removed.
- However, subsequent alterations in body contour may occur as a result of aging, weight gain or loss, and pregnancy.

ARE THERE ALTERNATIVES TO AN ABDOMINOPLASTY?

- Dieting will reduce the fat, but the excess skin, stretch marks, and loose muscle will not be affected.
- Exercise may improve the muscle tone, but it will not affect the excess skin or stretch marks.
- Liposuction will remove the excess fat, but it will not affect the excess skin, stretch marks, or lax muscle.

WHO ARE GOOD CANDIDATES FOR AN ABDOMINOPLASTY?

- The best candidates are individuals who are in relatively good shape, but bothered by a significant amount of loose abdominal skin or fat that will not respond to diet or exercise.
- The surgery is especially helpful to women who have been pregnant and who have stretched their abdominal muscles and skin beyond the point at which they will return to normal.
- If you intend to lose a fair amount of weight relative to your size, you should postpone all body-contouring surgery until after the weight loss.
- Women who plan future pregnancies are encouraged to wait until they have had all of their children. The abdominal muscles are tightened during surgery and will separate with pregnancy.

24

Arm Lift (Bracheoplasty)

WHAT IS A BRACHEOPLASTY, AND WHAT DOES IT ACCOMPLISH?

- A bracheoplasty is a surgical procedure to remove excess skin and fatty tissue from the upper part of the arm, extending from the level of the underarm to the level of the elbow.
- Overweight individuals who intend to lose weight should postpone all forms of body-contouring surgery until they have lost the extra weight and have been able to maintain their new weight for at least six months.
- A bracheoplasty can be performed by itself or combined with other forms of body-contouring surgery, including liposuction.
- It improves the contour of the arm and provides a youthful, firmer appearance by removing the sagging tissue.

WHAT ARE THE LIMITATIONS OF A BRACHEOPLASTY?

- A bracheoplasty cannot completely eliminate loose skin and excess fat; it will improve the condition.
- The scar extends along the full length of the upper arm. It is placed along the inside of the arm so as to minimize its visibility, but it is permanent.
- Patients with very heavy arms may require liposuction of the arms as an initial separate procedure before a bracheoplasty can be safely and effectively performed.

HOW IS A BRACHEOPLASTY PERFORMED?

- The patient is marked with the arms extended away from the body.
- An ellipse of skin is outlined along the inner upper arm. This extends from just above the level of the elbow to the underarm region.
- The width of the ellipse of tissue to be removed is determined by the extent of sagging skin. The more tissue to be removed, the greater the width of the ellipse.
- Care is taken to ensure that there is a smooth contour from the level of the elbow extending all the way along the upper arm.
- After the excess tissue of both arms is measured to provide a good degree of symmetry, the patient proceeds to the operating room.
- The outlined ellipse of excess tissue is removed, and each arm is tightened by closing the incision using several layers of sutures.

DOES A BRACHEOPLASTY HURT?

- You will have some pain along the incisions. This is usually described as a sharp or burning sensation. Although everyone is different in terms of their pain tolerance, most patients report the pain as very mild.
- If the pain is more than can be managed by the prescribed medications, you need to notify your surgeon.

WHERE ARE THE SCARS FOLLOWING A BRACHEOPLASTY?

- For a regular bracheoplasty, the scar is along the full length of the inner aspect of the upper arm, extending from the elbow up to the underarm area.
- If a woman has a very limited amount of excess skin along the underarm area, a more limited procedure is performed, with a scar limited to the underarm area. The scar is usually hidden within the creases of skin and not easily seen. However, this is possible only in a limited number of individuals. This chapter will discuss the classic bracheoplasty.

WHAT KIND OF ANESTHESIA IS RECOMMENDED DURING A BRACHEOPLASTY?

- Most surgeons will recommend general anesthesia for a bracheoplasty.
- Twilight anesthesia (local anesthesia with sedation) may be also be used in certain cases, depending on the extent of surgery needed and the individual patient's degree of comfort.

WHAT CAN I EXPECT AFTER A BRACHEOPLASTY?

- When you awaken in the recovery room, you will be in a semi-sitting position with your arms slightly elevated (usually with a pillow under each arm).
- Some surgeons wrap the arms, beginning at the level of the wrist all the way up to the underarm area, with an Ace bandage. Others prefer the use of a garment to provide support and slight compression.
- Expect to feel slight tightness along the entire length of the upper arm. Also, you will experience a slight burning sensation along the incision.
- During the first week after a bracheoplasty, you would benefit from sleeping with a pillow under each arm to keep the arms in a slightly elevated position. This helps to decrease the degree of swelling, which helps with the healing process.
- Most patients do not have significant bruising following a bracheoplasty. If liposuction is performed in conjunction with a bracheoplasty, you should expect slightly more bruising.
- You will have some swelling along the entire arm after a bracheo-plasty. In cases of significant swelling immediately after surgery, patients may experience tingling in their fingertips. This needs to be reported to your surgeon immediately, since it indicates that there is compression along the nerves.
- It is normal to experience some swelling after surgery. Although much of this resolves after the first two weeks, there may be residual swelling for up to 6–12 months, depending on the degree of the surgery.
- You should expect to have numbness along the incision and adjacent skin. This numbness improves over time. You may feel

slight tingling along the arm, as the nerves are healing from surgery. Sensation returns to most of the arm, but some numbness may be permanent.

- You will appreciate a significant difference in the contour of your arms immediately after surgery. However, it may take approximately three months before you will see most of the results, and it can take up to one year before you see the complete effect.

HOW DO I CARE FOR MYSELF AFTER A BRACHEOPLASTY?

- The incisions will usually be covered with surgical tape (Steri-strips). The tape should be left in place until it falls off by itself or is removed in your surgeon's office.
- If you were placed in a support garment, you should remove it only to shower until your surgeon advises you that you no longer need to wear it.
- Starting the day after surgery, you should walk at home as much as you can comfortably tolerate.
- You may begin activities of daily living, such as brushing your teeth, washing your face, showering, and getting dressed, immediately after your surgery.
- Most patients do not experience significant pain following a bracheoplasty. Although you will be given prescription pain medication, you may change to Tylenol within a couple of days after surgery.
- When lying in bed for the first week, use one pillow under each arm. This keeps your arms elevated, decreasing the swelling during the initial healing period.
- You may resume light household duties that do not require lifting and pulling/pushing within a few days after surgery.
- You should not drive until you are off all prescription pain medication.
- It will take approximately two weeks until you feel like you are moving your arms freely.
- Since you will not have normal sensation along the upper arms immediately after surgery, you should not use hot-water bottles or heating pads, as you may burn the skin.
- You should refrain from tanning and tanning beds for at least six weeks. The actual incisions should not be tanned until they are

completely healed and faded. This is usually after the first one or two years. If a scar is exposed to the sun or to a tanning bed while it is still red or pink, it will become dark and potentially remain that way long term.

- You should limit excessive use of your arms during the first two weeks. You should also avoid lifting anything heavier than five pounds during the first two weeks after surgery and 20 pounds during the first three months after surgery, since this may strain the repair and lead to widening of your scar.

- The time required before you can safely return to work depends upon the extent of lifting and upper arm strain that your job demands.

- Although you are encouraged to walk immediately after surgery, you should not participate in any exercise regimen that requires great usage of your arms (such as tennis) until given clearance by your surgeon.

- The incision may become a little raised in some areas, but this will settle down in time.

HOW LONG WILL THE EFFECT OF A BRACHEOPLASTY LAST?

- The effect of the bracheoplasty should last for years, since the excess skin and fat are removed.

- However, as subsequent alterations in body contour occur as a result of aging and weight gain or loss, you should expect the arms to also change. With aging and following weight loss, there will be relaxation of the skin, and additional sagging will occur.

WHO ARE GOOD CANDIDATES FOR A BRACHEOPLASTY?

- The best candidates are individuals who are in relatively good shape, but bothered by a significant amount of loose upper-arm skin or fat that will not respond to diet or exercise.

- The surgery is especially helpful to women who have lost a great deal of weight and whose skin has been stretched beyond the point that it will return to normal.

- If you intend to lose a significant amount of weight relative to your size, you should postpone any body-contouring surgery until after the weight loss.

- Patients contemplating a bracheoplasty should begin an exercise regimen to improve the muscle tone along the upper arms prior to surgery. This not only improves the blood supply to the area thereby enhancing healing, but it also improves the contour of the arms.

HOW LONG WILL THE EFFECT OF A BRACHEOPLASTY LAST?

- Like all other body-contouring procedures, the effect of a bracheo-plasty is dependent upon the patient's weight and exercise regimen after surgery. Significant weight gain or loss will decrease the improvement seen after surgery. Those who maintain their weight without major fluctuations and continue their exercise regimen should expect long-term improvement of their arms.
- Just as aging affects the skin of the face, it also affects the skin along the rest of the body. Keep in mind that inner-arm skin, like the inner-thigh skin, is much thinner than the skin along other parts of the body. Consequently, it manifests the signs of aging faster. As the individual ages, the contour of the arms following bracheoplasty will not be as tight.

ARE THERE ALTERNATIVES TO A BRACHEOPLASTY?

- Liposuction may be a surgical alternative to bracheoplasty if there is good skin tone and localized fatty deposits in an individual of normal weight.
- Diet and exercise programs may be of benefit in the overall reduction of excess body fat, but will not improve the excess skin.

25

Thigh Lift

WHAT IS A THIGH LIFT?

- A thigh lift is a surgical procedure to remove excess skin and fat from the upper part of the thigh.
- A thigh lift is not a surgical treatment for being overweight. Overweight individuals who intend to lose weight should postpone all forms of body-contouring surgery until they have reached their goal weight and have been able to maintain their weight loss for at least six months.
- In certain cases, a thigh lift may be combined with other forms of body-contouring surgery, including liposuction.

WHAT DOES A THIGH LIFT ACCOMPLISH?

- By removing the excess skin and fat from the upper part of the thigh, a thigh lift effectively addresses the upper one-half to two-thirds of the thigh to provide a firmer, thinner appearance.
- With time, the skin and soft tissues along the thigh lose their firmness. This is especially true along the inner thigh, but may occur along the outer thigh as well. These effects are more pronounced in individuals who have lost a significant amount of weight. The increased skin laxity creates a rippled appearance along the thigh.
- By lifting the skin and removing the extra skin and fat, the thigh has a smoother appearance with a better contour.

WHAT ARE THE LIMITATIONS OF A THIGH LIFT?

- A thigh lift cannot remove excess skin and fat without a noticeable scar.
  - In the majority of cases of inner thigh laxity, the scar is placed within the groin along the inner thigh crease (where the thigh meets the hip), making it less visible.
  - In cases of outer thigh laxity, the incision is placed along the outer hip, extending towards the pubic region and the back, depending upon the extent of the excess skin to be removed.
  - In cases of severe excess skin and laxity, the incision may be placed along the full length of the inner part of the thigh, extending from the level of the groin to just above the knee. This approach is reserved for cases of severe laxity, as the scar is not easily hidden.
- A thigh lift cannot eliminate stretch marks unless they are in the segment of skin that is removed.
- It is not permanent. The laxity of the skin increases over time, and gravity continues to affect the tissues on a daily basis.
- As gravity takes its toll, the position of the incision may change. If the incision is placed at the level of the groin within the inner upper thigh crease, it may shift down with time. This will make the scar more visible and often necessitates revision.

HOW IS A THIGH LIFT PERFORMED?

- The patient is marked in the upright standing position to determine the amount of skin to remove from the upper inner thigh, the outer thigh, or along the entire length of the inner thigh without excessive strain on the closure. This is outlined with a marker. The remainder of the thigh is evaluated to determine if liposuction needs to be performed along the tissues of the thigh that are not lifted in order to obtain a better contour. These are similarly marked with the patient in standing position.
- If needed, liposuction is usually performed first along the fuller areas of the thigh. The skin and soft tissues are then elevated from the underlying muscle layer, and the excess skin and soft tissues are removed. The two edges of tissue are then sewn together to provide a lift and improve the contour.
- The muscles are not altered with a thigh lift procedure.

WHAT IS THE RECOVERY TIME FOLLOWING A THIGH LIFT?

- Depending on the extensiveness of the thigh lift, most patients require approximately one to two weeks following surgery before resuming work and most normal daily activities.

DOES A THIGH LIFT HURT?

- Most patients complain of discomfort with movement following a thigh lift. This lasts approximately two to three days following surgery. After this period of time, the majority of patients use non-narcotic medications for pain management.

WHAT KIND OF ANESTHESIA IS RECOMMENDED DURING A THIGH LIFT?

- Although some plastic surgeons will use twilight anesthesia, the majority of plastic surgeons recommend general anesthesia for a thigh lift.

WHAT CAN I EXPECT AFTER A THIGH LIFT?

- When you awaken in the recovery room, you will have a wrapping along the full length of each leg extending from the level of the ankle to the level of the upper thigh. This is intended to provide a slight compression and support the legs.
- There will be mild-to-moderate aching along the areas that underwent liposuction as well as a burning-type pain along the incision lines.
- Your legs will be checked for normal blood flow to the feet during the first few hours after surgery. This is performed to ensure that the wrappings are not too tight and that the procedure did not compromise the blood supply along the legs.
- You should expect some swelling and bruising along the thighs. Both are worse at two days after surgery than they are immediately following surgery.

- With walking, the bruising and swelling gravitate down toward the lower legs. This is normal, and elevating the legs helps alleviate the symptoms.

- You may experience twinges of sharp pain along the incisions due to the nerves healing from surgery. This improves with time.

- As you heal, expect some numbness along the thighs and the incisions. Although the majority of this improves over the course of the first six months, some numbness may be permanent.

HOW DO I CARE FOR MYSELF AFTER A THIGH LIFT?

- Most surgeons use some type of supportive dressing during the first week after surgery. Many prefer wrapping the legs in an Ace wrap to provide support. This should be worn from the level of the ankle to the level of the upper thigh at all times except when showering.

- Some surgeons prefer a girdle-type garment along the full length of the leg for adequate support. After the first week, you may begin wearing support pantyhose.

- You are encouraged to walk as soon as possible after surgery so as to decrease the risk of a blood clot forming in the major leg veins. However, standing for a long period of time immediately after surgery is discouraged, since it will increase swelling along the legs. Starting the day after surgery, you should get up and walk inside the house several times per day.

- The incisions are usually covered with surgical tape (Steri-strips), which should remain in place until advised by your surgeon. The tape helps protect the incision during the early period after surgery. Most surgeons will remove the tape after two weeks.

- When lying in bed, you may be more comfortable by placing pillows under your knees and behind your back. This helps to decrease the tension along the incision. Also, when lying on your side, it often helps to keep a small pillow in between your knees.

- Do not drive until you are free of pain, feel comfortable, and are off all pain medication.

- The incision may be slow to heal. Once the tape is removed, you may clean the incisions once or twice daily with soap and water.

- Do not use ice compresses, hot-water bottles, or heating pads until all sensation returns to the thighs.

- You should not use a tub, whirlpool, or swimming pool until given clearance by your surgeon.
- You should avoid tanning and tanning beds until all bruising has resolved and the incisions have faded. If the incisions are exposed to the sun or to tanning beds while they are still red or pink, the scar will become darker in color and may remain discolored permanently.
- You may resume sexual intercourse four to six weeks after surgery or when comfortable enough to do so.
- Please refrain from any type of thigh exercises beyond walking until further instructed by your surgeon. Activities such as jogging, bicycling, swimming, etc., can potentially place too much stress along your thigh lift incisions.

HOW LONG WILL THE EFFECT OF A THIGH LIFT LAST?

- Like most body-lifting procedures, the long-term effects of a thigh lift depend upon the quality of the individual's skin as well as subsequent changes in the person's weight and exercise regimen.
- If there are significant changes with weight gain followed by weight loss, the laxity will surely return at a faster rate than when the individual maintains a constant reasonable weight with a healthy exercise regimen.

ARE THERE ALTERNATIVES TO A THIGH LIFT?

- Liposuction may be a surgical alternative to a thigh lift in a limited number of cases if there is good skin tone and localized fatty deposits in individuals of normal weight.
- Diet and exercise programs may be of benefit in the overall reduction of excess body fat.

WHO ARE GOOD CANDIDATES FOR A THIGH LIFT?

- Individuals who have lost significant amounts of weight, or who have undergone liposuction of the thighs with resulting poor skin retraction, as well as those with genetically lax skin may benefit from a thigh lift.

26

Labial Reduction (Labiaplasty)

WHAT IS A LABIAPLASTY?

- Labiaplasty is a surgical procedure to treat enlarged or asymmetrical labia minora (external folds of skin surrounding the vaginal opening).
- It is also called labia minor reduction or labial reduction.
- It may be performed on one or both sides of the labia minora.
- The procedure reduces and reshapes the labia minora by removing the excess and often discolored tissue in order to provide a more symmetrical refined appearance.
- Significant enlargement of the labia minora may be due to genetic or hormonal reasons. It may also develop after injury, sexual intercourse, childbirth, and aging.
- Women seek this procedure for functional or aesthetic reasons, or a combination of the two.
- Labiaplasty may be of benefit for women who experience discomfort and chafing during sexual or sports activities if due to enlarged labia minora.

HOW IS A LABIAPLASTY PERFORMED?

- The patient is marked in the frog-leg position to determine the amount of tissue to remove from the labia minora while still maintaining an adequate rim of tissue.

- The excess tissue is removed, and the remaining tissue is re-positioned to create a natural smaller and more aesthetic labia minora.
- At times, some of the tissue along the clitoral hood (tissue covering the clitoris) needs to be removed.
- Care must be taken to ensure that the exact, proper amount of tissue is removed. Excessive tissue removal may result in tissue distortion, tissue dryness, unacceptable appearance, or excessive pulling. If excessive tissue is removed from the clitoral hood, there may be increased sensitivity.
- If needed, liposuction may be performed along the mons pubis to decrease any fullness in that area to obtain a better contour.

WHEN IS THE RIGHT TIME TO CONSIDER A LABIAPLASTY?

- It is important to ensure that the labia are completely developed prior to considering surgery.
- Performing a labiaplasty prior to complete sexual development may only create the need for additional surgery in the future.
- Often, pregnancy and childbirth will result in an enlargement the labia minora. If a woman has decided to undergo the procedure after having a child, it is better to wait until she has finished having children.

DOES A LABIAPLASTY HURT?

- Although there is some discomfort along the incision, the pain is easily controlled with the prescribed pain medication.
- Most patients complain of slight discomfort with movement or periods of prolonged sitting during the first few days after surgery.
- In general, this is not considered a very painful procedure.

WHAT KIND OF ANESTHESIA IS RECOMMENDED DURING A LABIAPLASTY?

- Depending on the extensiveness of the procedure and the patient's comfort level, different types of anesthesia may be used. If the procedure is minor, it may be performed under local anesthesia. If it is more extensive, the majority of plastic surgeons recommend either twilight or general anesthesia.

WHAT ARE SOME OF THE LONG-TERM EFFECTS OF A LABIAPLASTY?

- In general, the changes achieved with labial reduction surgery are expected to be permanent.
- However, subsequent alterations in the labia tissues may occur as the result of aging, weight loss or gain, pregnancy, or other circumstances not related to labiaplasty surgery.

WHAT CAN I EXPECT AFTER A LABIAPLASTY?

- When you awaken in the recovery area, you will feel a slight burning pain along the incisions.
- Although there is some discomfort during the first few days, it is easily controlled with the prescribed pain medication.
- You should expect to have some mild swelling and bruising in the area. However, if you experience pain with significant bruising and swelling, it may represent internal bleeding and should be reported to your surgeon immediately.
- Voiding may be slightly uncomfortable in the first day or two after surgery. This is due to the tissue inflammation from surgery and swelling along the area.
- Prolonged walking and sitting will be uncomfortable during the first few days.
- You may experience twinges of pain, as the nerves are healing from surgery.
- Some women report increased sensitivity along the labia minora after the healing process is complete.
- There is the potential for numbness along the labia due to cutting some of the nerves, but this is rare.

HOW DO I TAKE CARE OF MYSELF AFTER A LABIAPLASTY?

- You may shower the day after surgery.
- You may use ice compresses during the first few days for comfort. Ice should not be applied directly to the area; instead, it should be applied through a thin cloth to ensure comfort.

- During the first week after surgery, it is important to keep the incisions clean. You may do so by showering or by briefly soaking in a bathtub once or twice daily.
- The incisions may be covered with an ointment like Aquaphor to help with the discomfort and with wound healing.
- For the first week after surgery, you may experience slight pink drainage and minimal bleeding along the incisions. Non-adherent gauze should be worn for comfort.
- When lying in bed, you may find it helpful to keep your legs bent with a pillow under the knees, as this alleviates some of the discomfort. When lying on one side, you may keep a small pillow between your knees to serve the same purpose.
- You may resume sexual intercourse six weeks after surgery when it becomes comfortable to do so.
- You should avoid jogging, bicycling, swimming, contact sports, or any aerobic or non-aerobic activity that places pressure on the surgical area for the first four to six weeks.

WHAT IS THE RECOVERY TIME FOLLOWING A LABIAPLASTY?

- Depending on the extensiveness of the labiaplasty, most patients require approximately five to seven days following surgery to feel comfortable resuming work and normal daily activities.
- Full recovery usually takes two to three months.

Plastic Surgery in the Future

27

Advances in Plastic Surgery

The last decade has witnessed tremendous advances in plastic surgery. There is an obviously greater acceptance of plastic surgery worldwide. Some may say it is more than an acceptance, but rather an encouragement. Some may even say that plastic surgery has created a new "normal." Have we in fact changed the norm? What does the future hold? Will having a disproportionate nose or prominent frown lines be socially unacceptable in the future? Will this have significant implications for the success of personal relationships and professional careers? We have seen from many psychological experiments that attractive people are viewed more favorably under nearly all circumstances. Will the inability or unwillingness to change one's "less desirable" features be seen as a flaw in itself? Do we have a subconscious or hard-wired understanding and acceptance of the "what is beautiful is good" principle? The desire to improve our appearance seems to be a very natural intrinsic trait.

With a greater awareness of what can be achieved through invasive and noninvasive procedures, we are seeing a desire for less invasive procedures being performed at an earlier point in life. Younger people are seeking procedures to enhance and maintain their youthful appearance, rather than waiting until their features age. As we attempt to preserve youth, we are becoming "ageless." It is increasingly difficult to determine someone's biological age based on their physical appearance. Initially, the trend in plastic surgery shifted from repair of age-related changes to maintenance of youthful features, and now maintenance is paving the way to prevention of the aging process. This is most notable with the use of Botox Cosmetic to prevent frown lines and crow's feet, and potentially minimize the need for a surgical brow lift. Similarly, use of soft tissue fillers in the lips to maintain a healthy fullness prevents or minimizes the fine wrinkles around the lips ("smoker's lines").

As plastic surgery continues to flourish, we will witness great improvements in various products and procedures. Breast implants are expected to become more customized based on the patient's anatomy. Greater options in soft tissue fillers will become available, allowing for longer-lasting correction of facial aging. Tissue-tightening lasers will become increasingly more advanced and will be expected to create more remarkable results with less downtime. More advanced liposuction procedures will allow better skin retraction following fat removal, and consequently, better results. Less invasive surgical facial rejuvenation procedures will allow more of these cases to be performed with patients fully awake, and consequently, allow a greater safety measure.

The most fascinating prospect in the future of plastic surgery is the role of stem cells. Stem-cell research is providing a glimpse of the possibility of not just repairing our organs, but actually regenerating new tissues. Stem cells are found in all multicellular organisms. They are characterized by their ability to regenerate themselves and differentiate into specialized cell types. The two main types of stem cells in humans are embryonic stem cells found in embryos (blastocytes), and adult stem cells found in adult tissues.

The embryonic stem cells can differentiate into all of the specialized tissues: heart, kidneys, lungs, skin, bones, muscles, nerves, etc. The adult stem cells repair and maintain tissues that undergo significant turnover, such as skin and intestinal tissues. Stem cells can be grown and transformed into cells having the characteristics of specialized tissues such as muscles and nerves. Currently, adult stem cells from bone marrow and umbilical cord blood are used in various medical treatments.

If stem cells allow for regeneration of our tissues, we will be able to reverse damaged tissues in every organ in our body: Damaged heart muscle will be replaced with healthy muscle; damaged kidneys will be replaced with functioning ones; and aged tissue will be replaced with its youthful counterpart. Indeed, we are on the verge of stepping into the fountain of youth.

Although plastic surgery may not add years to your life, it is my sincerest wish that it adds much life to your years.

Appendix

Medications, Herbs, Supplements, and Other Substances to Avoid Prior to Surgery

Medications That Increase the Risk of Bleeding during Surgery

Acetidine	Aspercin	Clinoril
Advil	Aspirin	Codoxy
Aleve	Axotal	Congesprin
Alka-Seltzer	Azolid	Coricidin
Anacin	Bayer	Cosprin
Anahist	Bromo-Seltzer	Darvon ASA
Anaprox	Buffaprin	Diclofenac
Anexsia	Bufferin	Diflusanal
Ansaid	Buffex	Dipyridamole
Anturane	Buffinol	Doan's Pills
Arthritis Bayer	Butazolidin	Dolcin
Arthritis Pain Formula	Butazone	Dolene Compound
Ascriptin	Cama	Dolobid
Asper Buf	Celebrex	Dristan

(Continues)

The risks and benefits of additional medications, herbs, and supplements are continuously being discovered. As such, this list is not all-inclusive. Be certain to discuss all products that you ingest with your surgeon prior to your surgery. Furthermore, do not resume taking any of these drugs following surgery until cleared by your surgeon.

Duragesic	Lodine	Pabirin
Easprin	Lortab ASA	Pepto-Bismol
Ecotrin	Magnaprin	Percodan
Efficin	Magsal	Persantine
Emagrin	Maprin	Persistin
Empirin	Mejoral	Phenybutazone
Equagesic	Mefanamic Acid	Presalin
Equazine-M	Mepro-Analgesic	Relafen
Etodolac	Methacin	Rufen
Excedrin	Micrainin	Saleto
Feldene	Midol	Salocol
Fenoprofen	Mobidin	SK-65 Compound
Fiorinal	Mobigesic	Sulindac
Flubiprofen	Monogesic	Synalgos
Gaysal-S	Motrin	Talwin
Gemnisyn	Nabumetone	Tandearil
Goody's Headache	Nalfon	Tenstan
Powder	Naprosyn	Theracin
Ibuprofen	Naproxen	Tolectin
Indocin	Neocylate	Tolmetin
Indomethacin	Norgesic	Toradol
Inhiston	Nuprin	Trigesic
Isollyl	Orudis	Vanquish
Ketoprofen	Oruvail	Voltaren
Ketorolac	Oxalid	Zoprin
Lanorinal	Oxyphenbutazone	

If a medical doctor has prescribed any of the drugs on this list, you must notify that doctor prior to stopping the medication.
http://www.pdrhealth.com (accessed January 3, 2010)

Herbs and Supplements That Increase the Risk of Bleeding during Surgery

Acai	Celery*	Ginkgo
Agrimony	Chondroitin	Ginseng
Alfalfa*	Clove	Glucosamine
Angelica	Danshen	Goldenseal
Anise*	Dong Quai	Horse Chestnut
Asafoetida	European Mistletoe	Horseradish
Aspen	Fenugreek	Licorice*
Black Cohosh	Feverfew	Meadowsweet
Bog bean	Fish Oil	Northern Prickly Ash
Boldo	Flaxseed Oil	Onion*
Borage Seed Oil	Fucus	Papain
Bromelain	Garlic*	Passion Flower
Capsicum	Ginger*	Pau D'arco

Plantain	St. Johns Wort	Wild Carrot*
Poplar	Stinging Nettle	Wild Lettuce*
Quassia	Sweet Clover	Willow Bark
Red Clover	Sweet Vernal Grass	Yarrow
Roman Chamomile	Tonka Bean	
Safflower*	Turmeric	
Southern Prickly Ash	Vitamin E*	

*These herbs may be consumed in the form of ordinary foods, but not in any supplement form (pills, liquids, powders, energy bars, specialty teas, etc.).

PDR for Herbal Medicines, 2nd ed. Montvale, NJ: Medical Economics Company, Inc., 2000.

G. Broughton II et al. "Use of Herbal Supplements and Vitamins in Plastic Surgery: A Practical Review." *Plastic and Reconstructive Surgery Journal*. 2007. 48e–66e.

J. Heller et al. "Top-10 List of Herbal and Supplemental Medicines Used by Cosmetic Patients: What the Plastic Surgeon Needs to Know." *Plastic and Reconstructive Surgery Journal*. 2006. 436–45.

Substances That Compromise Wound Healing following Surgery

Tobacco
Nicotine Patches
Nicotine Gum

P. Silverstein. "Smoking and Wound Healing" *American Journal of Medicine*. 1992; 93 (1A): 22s–24s.

K. Knobloch et al. "Nicotine in Plastic Surgery: A Review." (Article in German) *Chirurg*. 2008; 79 (10): 956–62.

Notes

Introduction

1. Merriam-Webster Online, http://www.merriamwebster.com/dictionary/vanity (accessed September 29, 2009).

2. American Society for Aesthetic Plastic Surgery, *Cosmetic Surgery National Data Bank Statistics* (2007).

3. American Society for Aesthetic Plastic Surgery, *Cosmetic Surgery National Data Bank Statistics* (2008).

4. Ibid.

5. Ibid.

6. Ibid.

7. Ibid.

8. Ibid.

9. Ibid.

10. American Society for Aesthetic Plastic Surgery, *Cosmetic Surgery National Data Bank Statistics* (2007).

11. American Society for Aesthetic Plastic Surgery, *Cosmetic Surgery National Data Bank Statistics* (2008).

Chapter 2: Beauty in History and Its Social Impact

1. Aristotle Quotations Online, http://www.quotationspage.com/quotes/Aristotle (accessed September 28, 2009).

2. Merriam-Webster Online, http://www.merriamwebster.com/dictionary/icon (accessed September 29, 2009).

3. K. Dion, et al. "What Is Beautiful Is Good." *Journal of Personality and Social Psychology* 1972. Vol. 24(3), 285–290.

4. Nancy Etcoff. *Survival of the Prettiest: The Science of Beauty.* New York, NY: Doubleday, 1999.
5. Ibid.

Chapter 4: Body Dysmorphic Disorder

1. K. A. Phillips, *The Broken Mirror: Understanding and Treating Body Dysmorphic Disorder.* New York, NY: Oxford University Press, 1996.
2. Ibid.
3. "ASAPS Members Answer Questions about BDD." *Aesthetic Society News.* Vol 5(3), 15. October 23, 2001.
4. Ibid.
5. Phillips.
6. "ASAPS Members Answer Questions."
7. Phillips.
8. Ibid.
9. Ibid.
10. Ibid.
11. Ibid.
12. Ibid.
13. Ibid.

Chapter 5: Plastic Surgery and Adolescents

1. American Society of Plastic Surgeons. *2009 Report of the 2008 Statistics.* National Clearinghouse of Plastic Surgery Statistics.

Chapter 7: Preparing for Your Surgery

1. *PDR for Herbal Medicines,* 2nd ed. Montvale, NJ: Medical Economics Company, Inc., 2000.
2. Ibid.
3. Ibid.

Chapter 21: Breast Reduction in Men (Gynecomastia Surgery)

1. *Grabb and Smith's Plastic Surgery,* 4th ed. Little, Brown and Company, 1991.

Index

About the Author

ILIANA E. SWEIS, MD, FACS, is a board-certified plastic surgeon and fellow of the American College of Surgeons. She is clinical assistant professor of surgery at the University of Illinois at Chicago and a member of the Board of Directors of the Illinois Society of Plastic Surgeons. Dr. Sweis completed her training in plastic surgery at Northwestern University School of Medicine. Her experience and skill have earned her many distinguished honors, including being selected on numerous occasions as one of the top plastic surgeons in the country by the Consumers' Research Council of America. She is also founder and president of the Royal Service Children's Foundation, an organization sponsored and supported by the late King Hussein of Jordan, which has led medical missions to the Middle East to perform surgery on those in need. Dr. Sweis has been in private practice since 1997 and focuses exclusively on surgical and non-surgical facial rejuvenation, breast enhancement, and body contouring. She practices in Northbrook, Illinois, and in downtown Chicago.